WHAT IF TODAY'S CHOICES COULD TRANSFORM YOUR HEALTH—AND YOUR FUTURE?

After struggling with health issues for years, I discovered the power of evidence-based lifestyle changes. Improved blood markers, vanished symptoms, and newfound energy transformed my life. Now, I share my journey, essential health insights, and a practical, science-backed roadmap in *'The Complete Guide to Sustainable Health and Weight'*.

Discover:

- How to improve gut health, reduce inflammation, and boost vitality.
- A behavioral science-based plan to build healthy habits, achieve lasting weight loss, and maintain sustainable progress.
- Insights into fibers, proteins, fats, and other critical elements of balanced nutrition.
- A sustainable, no-extreme-restrictions approach to eating and living.

This guide bridges the gap between complex science and everyday life. It includes a practical behavioral model designed to help you embrace healthier habits, lose weight, and keep it off—empowering you to reclaim your energy and well-being.

Whether you're aiming to lose weight, prevent disease, or enhance your longevity, this book equips you with the tools to take control of your health and build a sustainable future.

THE COMPLETE GUIDE TO A SUSTAINABLE HEALTH AND WEIGHT

MASTER DIET, EXERCISE, AND BEHAVIOR FOR
LONG-TERM WELLNESS AND LONGEVITY

MAGNUS BENGTSSON

COPYRIGHT

To **Rose**, *my soulmate.*

Thank you for always supporting me.

Thank you for your valuable proofreading.

Thank you for your continuous encouragement.

Thank you for joining me on my health journey.

Thank you for your love.

INTRODUCTION

What you are probably most interested in knowing is - WHAT POSITIVE EFFECTS DO YOU GET WHEN YOU CHANGE YOUR LIFESTYLE?

One of my absolute favorite words is described by the Swedish Academy's dictionary as 'discomfort etc. that results from a course of action'. The reason I like the word is that it has a clear meaning. The word is 'Consequence'. Every time we make a choice, take a decision or perform an action, there is a consequence. It can be both immediate or further down the line. Whenever it is, we can be sure that at some point the results of our decisions will show up - as something good or something bad!

With this book, I want to give you the very best conditions to make good decisions.

In his poem **'Black Postcards'**, Tomas Tranströmer (Nobel Prize in Literature 2011) thoughtfully describes

how we live our lives without thinking about the consequences:

"In the middle of life, death comes and takes the measure of man. That visit is forgotten and life goes on. But the suit is sewn in silence."

It is described in the chapter 'About the Author' why I made my lifestyle change. To summarise it briefly - I had two choices, either to live as I did or to do a radical change. For me, the decision was easy - I wanted to stick around for a while longer and I wanted to be in control of my life.

My cholesterol was way too high and it was killing me. It was fixed and I was put on medication. But medication alone didn't solve the problem so I decided to cut off all cholesterol intake (the body makes its own cholesterol but we also eat food that contains cholesterol). This means stop eating meat because only animal foods contain cholesterol. Said and done, I became completely plant-based 5 years ago. Back then, when I didn't have the knowledge I have today, I assumed that all vegan food is healthy. It definitely is not. Many vegan foods are ultra-processed and contain unhealthy additives. So be careful what you buy.

But don't get me wrong - you are welcome to continue eating meat. This book is not a rule book with pointers but a book of knowledge from which you can choose parts that suit you and your way of life. But if you have high cholesterol or ongoing inflammation in your body, then you should reduce the amount of meat you eat.

Nowadays, I eat mostly unprocessed, fresh vegetables that I prepare.

Positive effects of my lifestyle change

(I only eat a plant-based diet including time-restricted eating):

I used to be very tired after one or two nights of poor sleep.

Today I never feel tired after nights with less sleep.

In the past, when I caught a cold, I had a prolonged cough. It was not uncommon for it to last for a couple of months and sometimes that happened both in autumn and spring.

Today, when I catch a cold, I rarely cough for longer than 1 to 2 weeks.

In the past I had a couple of kilos overweight and had difficulty reaching my desired weight.

Today I have no problem maintaining my ideal weight. Even if I gain a few kilos, it is easy to get back to my target weight.

In the past, when I ate everything, including lunch, my blood sugar fluctuated up and down and I often felt hungry.

Today, when I don't eat lunch (time-restricted eating), my blood sugar is at a stable level and I don't feel hungry in the middle of the day.

In the past, it was not uncommon for me to be constipated.

Today, my stomach works perfectly almost always.

In the past, I used to have frequent heartburn and had to take H2-blockers.

Today, I very rarely have heartburn and when I do, it is always connected to the fact that I ate or drank something I should avoid.

In the past, the circulation in my right foot (red-blue colored and cold) was reduced and that was one reason why I stopped snus 15 years ago. There was no improvement and neither when I started medication with statins 12 years ago.

Today, after diet change, the foot has regained its normal color and temperature.

In the past, I could not reach the target value for LDL cholesterol despite maximum dose statins.

Today the values are lower than before. Because of a family history of high cholesterol, I dare not stop taking the medication.

In the past I used to have problems with my back because I have cartilage formation between the vertebrae and ribs that makes me stiff.

Today my back is much better and the stiffness has disappeared. My back problems were probably aggravated by the inflammatory diet I used to eat.

In the past, I felt that my body couldn't keep up with my movements and I felt old and clumsy, for example when I went down stairs.

Today I can run down the stairs like when I was young.

And another not entirely unimportant detail worth mentioning - I used to be unable to walk past a candy store without getting a craving. After I stopped eating sweets, it only took a month or so before the craving disappeared. Today I don't feel any cravings when I pass a candy store. It became very clear how strong the sugar addiction is, but also that it is not that difficult to break. What helped me was the knowledge of the microbiota and that it is destroyed by ultra-processed products - like candy - and when on the one hand I am building a strong microbiota, then I don't want to break it down by eating sweets. This was pure knowledge that led to a consequence action.

I want to emphasize that all these improvements did not happen overnight. Some changes I noticed quite quickly, for others it has taken 4-5 years before it happened. And probably I will also discover new improvements in the future. Remember to be patient and don't look for quick fixes and immediate radical effects. If you want a healthy long life, there is not short cuts, only hard work based on knowledge.

Feedback after dietary advice from a person with Crohns disease (inflammatory bowel disease):

"You will forever be remembered as the person who changed my life. Your insights on diet, and the dietary advice related to my Crohn's disease, and how you motivated me to change my diet, completely changed my life. I have talked to many other people about my disease but you were more convincing."

We all have a wish that when we retire we will be healthy, and able to spend time with our grandchildren, travel and experience the world. But for that wish to come true, it takes a bit of preparation. And that goes for everybody.

If you want to be a happy and healthy retiree who can do all the things you want, this is what you have to do:

- Start saving early for your retirement. The longer you live, the more you want to do, the more money you need to set aside.
- If you want to grow old, you have to live healthy.

'Health' as a concept is difficult to define. Or actually, it's not. It's just an abstract word. Health is something you don't notice or appreciate until you lose it. You just take it for granted that it will be there. Until it's no longer there. And once you've lost it, chances are it's gone forever.

We are more familiar with diseases. The problem is that we think it's normal to get diseases when we get older. That everyone gets sick. But what does that have to do with being a healthy old person?

Most people are familiar with the concept of lifestyle diseases but find it difficult to make the connection between their lifestyle and why they get sick.

Healthy living is not something you do for a few weeks or months, it's something you do all the time. In other words, it is no different from living unhealthily. The contradiction is that living a healthy life is perceived as difficult, while living an unhealthy life seems very easy. It should be the other way round.

But wait a minute! What do you mean unhealthy? How do I know I am unhealthy? Well, that's the thing. That's what the

'$10,000 question' is all about. This guide goes through most of the dangers we as humans are exposed to, and what small adjustments we can make to turn around a slowly sinking ship. In a simple way. And all the advice is based on the latest science.

Be aware of the following:
You are responsible for your health.

You both play the lead role and direct the film about your life. And of course you want the movie about you to be a good movie with a happy ending.

We humans always compare ourselves to those who are worse off than 'me'. Those who smoke more, those who are more overweight, those who drink more alcohol, those who exercise less etc. Why is that? Maybe because we want to postpone a lifestyle change for a while longer. Even though we know deep down that it won't be easier to make the change next week. Quite the opposite.

If we take obesity as an example, it's well known that if your friends are overweight it increases the risk of you becoming overweight, compared to if your friends are of normal weight. Behavior is contagious.

If you socialize with someone who is more overweight than you are, you will appear less overweight yourself. But only when you are standing next to that person. Be aware of the danger of these kinds of comparisons.

I know it's hard to find the right knowledge on how to stay healthy. You find the information how to do it on the web, but it's hard to know what to look for, what information is reliable and what is not, to understand medical terminology etc.

This guide is based on the latest medical science on what you should and should not eat, how much you should exercise, what you should be aware of that is harmful in our environment etc. It is written in an understandable way. It explains how to implement these necessary changes in small steps and in the smoothest way possible. You will improve your knowledge a lot. Then it's up to you to decide how much you want to implement. But the simple equation is - the more health benefits you add and the more unhealthy you remove from your life, the more birthdays you will be able to celebrate.

What affects our health?

If I were to try to put a percentage on what factors affect our health, it might look like this (for most of us and most of the time):

Sedentary behavior 5%

Stress 5%

Sleep 5%

Chemicals, microplastics, air pollution 5%

Lifestyle (smoking, alcohol etc) 20%

Genes 10%

Diet 50%

These figures can off course differ between person and within a lifetime.

Most factors affect the gut microbiota (the billions of microorganisms in the gut), either in a negative or positive way. If we misbehave, it will cause a dysbiosis in the microbiota, which ultimately leads to disease. And conversely, if we boost the microbiota, we are more likely to be healthy.

A few words about our genes. You carry an inheritance that you received from your parents and your ancestors. Your genes are then mixed with your partner's when you have children and your combined genes are passed on to your children.

An important detail is that inheritance is not constant. Your ancestors lived in a way that influenced their genes. This may then be the reason why you suffer from certain diseases.

Today's society, with all the new harmful products such as microplastics, ultra-processed food and drink, air pollution, but also the way we cook our food (high temperature), is damaging our genes. This is likely to be a major factor in our illnesses and in young children suffering from serious diseases such as cancer.

It is not difficult to be healthy. The hard part is continuing to engage in unhealthy behavior, knowing that the consequences will affect me and everyone I care about. And for generations to come.

This book was originally written in Swedish and compiled manually by the author. It has since been translated into other languages with the help of AI. If there are misspellings or other errors, I apologize both from my side and from the AI.

THE BASICS OF HEALTH

Health is something abstract, something that everyone has heard of, something that most people take for granted but that no one realizes the importance of or appreciates until they have lost it.

CONTENTS

1

LONGEVITY

L ongevity is the term for a 'long and healthy life'.

Both governments and the medical profession have casually trumpeted the mantra that 'we are getting older'. At the same time, we are becoming increasingly overweight and suffering from diseases linked to obesity, such as type 2 diabetes, heart disease, cancer, etc. In October 2024, a study was published in Nature Aging, which followed the population between 1990-2019 (so that Covid would not affect the results) in rich countries. It was noted that life expectancy was slowing down.

And in the US, there is a 'shocking' decline in life expectancy starting in 2010 caused by diseases such as diabetes and heart disease in people aged around 40 to 60. And as many other countries tends to follow the US, the risk is that you will soon see the same trend in your country.

. . .

You may have heard of the 'blue zones' that are scattered around the world? These are areas with many healthy 100-year-olds (centenarians). Netflix has a 4-episode series called 'Blue Zones' where they visited these areas and investigated the correlations between people living in these zones.

Common factors were found to be

- they eat a lot of fruit, vegetables, legumes etc.
- they eat minimal meat and no processed products
- they stop eating when they are 80% full - in order to feel 80% full, you need to eat slowly as satiety signals only come after 20 minutes
- they do not smoke
- they exercise daily
- they drink alcohol in moderation
- they have a social network
- they do not stress
- they sleep well
- they have a daily activity that they look forward to doing and that makes it worth getting up in the morning

In short - they live a healthy life where a good outcome can be expected.

. . .

IF WE LOOK at our lives as an axis of time, it might be hard to see yourself at the end of that axis.

If you want to be healthy, live a long life and be able to do all the things you might have dreamed of doing when you retire, my advice is - look in the mirror. Take a long good look. Do you see a person who has the odds in their favor to become a healthy old person? If not, it's time you make a change. You can make it! And the sooner you start, the better outcome you have.

A CLARIFICATION, I have a negative and a positive message for you.

THE NEGATIVE MESSAGE is that if you are in your 40s and 50s and have an unhealthy life such as eating unhealthy, not exercising, smoking, drinking too much alcohol, being overweight etc, you are slowly heading for an untimely demise. You will become sick and frail and die prematurely. You will most likely suffer from one of the following diseases - heart disease, stroke, type 2 diabetes or cancer. And it's not a threat, it's a guarantee.

Being 70-75 years old, frail and using a walker is not a normal state or a coincidence, but a result of how we have lived our lives. It may seem unfair to say it, but it is a fact in the vast majority of cases. There are exceptions, of course. But hoping to be 'one in a million' not being affected by a bad lifestyle is probably hoping for too much.

THE POSITIVE MESSAGE is that if you change your lifestyle by modifying your diet, start exercising (you don't need to start running marathons), stop smoking, drink less alcohol, lose weight, you can get between 5-10 more healthy years of life, depending on how old you are when you make your change. You should take this offer seriously.

HERE ARE some studies that confirm these claims.

According to the results of a Norwegian study, a 40-year-old person who switched from an unhealthy diet to one that followed dietary recommendations of eating more whole grains, vegetables, fruit, fish and white meat, and less of red meat, processed meat, eggs, refined grains and sugary drinks, could increase their life expectancy by 9 years.

FOR A 70-YEAR-OLD MAN, the change would be equivalent to 4 years longer life and 4.4 years longer for a woman of the same age.

THIS STUDY also looked at which foods had the greatest impact on extending life. It found that more consumption of whole grains and nuts and less of red meat and sugary drinks were associated with the greatest improvements in life expectancy.

ANOTHER STUDY LOOKED at people who have genes that suggest they won't live as long, and found that healthy habits can extend your life.

· · ·

IF **YOU HAVE an unhealthy lifestyle** plus life-shortening genes, you are twice as likely to die prematurely compared to those who have good habits and do not have these genes.

According to the study, if people with life-shortening genes adopt healthy lifestyle habits instead, they can significantly offset their genetic risk of premature death.

Not smoking, physical activity, good sleep and good diet are the lifestyle factors that have the greatest impact on longevity and can reduce the effects of life-shortening genes by more than 60%.

THE **RESEARCHERS NOTED** that genes can influence the risk of dying from diseases such as cancer, heart disease and diabetes. However, people with a high genetic risk can extend their lives by almost 5.5 years by adopting a healthier lifestyle in their 40s.

PREVIOUSLY, it was assumed that our genes determined our longevity, but this study now paints a different picture.

Over 60 per cent of our fate is determined by factors that we can largely control ourselves: diet, exercise, smoking and sleep.

AFTER **CHANGING my lifestyle 5 years ago**, I can say that my health is significantly better than for the majority of 30-40 year olds. And I am over 60 years old. While of course I'm proud of that, it's quite sad to see how poor the health of younger people is.

· · ·

OTHER FACTORS that can affect our life expectancy are fasting. Today, there is a lot of research on aging and what is popular and used by almost all age researchers is intermittent fasting or time-restricted eating. Read more under Intermittent fasting.

What can be briefly mentioned is that this type of fasting affects some of our cells. When our cells get old, cell division stops and the cells die. But some cells become like zombies and are neither alive nor dead. These cells are called senescent cells and are thought to be a cause of our aging by secreting inflammatory substances into the body.

ANOTHER FACTOR that is also linked to aging and the onset of diseases is our telomeres. Telomeres are the 'sheaths' at the end of chromosomes (like the plastic on the ends of shoelaces) that protect our DNA (genes) from damage and have been linked to longevity. Telomeres are located in the outer part of each chromosome and contain no genes. Each time a cell divides, the chromosomes replicate and the telomeres shorten. This allows the cell to divide without losing vital genes. Eventually, the telomeres are too short for the cell to divide again and the cell ages or dies.

It has been found that a healthy diet consisting of legumes, whole grains, fresh fruit and vegetables, and exercise can extend the time it takes for telomeres to become short. Similarly, but in reverse, smoking, poor diet, alcohol, sedentary behavior, lack of sleep, stress, can accelerate the process of telomere shortening and thus accelerate our biological aging.

. . .

THE NATIONAL INSTITUTES OF HEALTH (NIH) recommends the following to promote healthy aging:

- exercise - according to one study, walking about 8,000 steps a day compared to 4,000 steps reduced mortality by 51%.
- eating a healthy diet, such as the Mediterranean diet, with plenty of fresh fruit and vegetables
- maintaining a healthy weight - exercise and a healthy diet help with this
- sleeping well
- not smoking, or if you are a smoker - stop smoking!
- limit your alcohol intake
- regular health check-ups
- taking care of your mental health and managing levels of stress

THERE IS a lot of research going on about our cells, both to get a better understanding of how they are involved in our aging, but there are also studies going on to try and extend our lives. Our best tools today for healthy aging are largely in our own hands. Through better diet, more exercise, less stress, not smoking, not drinking too much alcohol.

WHY DO WE MAKE UNHEALTHY DECISIONS?

Why do we make unhealthy decisions? Or bad decisions in general? This is how behavioral science explains it.

IF WE SET goals that we really want to achieve, it makes sense to break down a larger goal into smaller sub-goals. Instead of aiming for 12 kg of weight loss as a final goal, it's a bit easier to lose 1 kg per month. Of course, after 1 year, 12 kg is still the final goal, but the journey is not as difficult when you strive to achieve the small sub-goals. All changes take time. All changes must also be sustainable over time. Accept that instead of investing in unsustainable quick fixes.

If you are going to change your diet, it is better to introduce 1 or 2 new ingredients and remove as many in the first stage and then repeat the procedure with 1-2 new changes once the routine of the first ones has set in.

. . .

To do this, we need to understand how our brain works to make decisions - to understand how we process information and on what basis we make decisions.

Two decision-making systems:

Daniel Kahneman (1934-2024), was a professor of psychology and behavioral science and was awarded the Nobel Prize in Economics in 2002 for his research on our decision-making systems. He called these systems 1 and 2. To better understand the meaning of each system, we can call them the Automatic and Reflective systems.

The Automatic system (System 1) - reaction when someone throws a ball at you, your reaction to air pits, smiling when you see something nice, driving a car, all the routine tasks you perform in your everyday life. Habits are also governed by the Automatic System. This system is associated with the oldest parts of the brain - the reptilian brain.

The Reflective System (System 2) - is more calculating and self-conscious. This system is used when you let your mind take a second turn before making decisions, when learning to do complicated things like driving a car.

One of the main tasks of the Reflective System is to monitor and control the thoughts and actions suggested by the Automatic System. Some of this is accepted, passed on and manifested in our behavior, while others are withheld or modified.

. . .

If the reflective system is so much better for us, why don't we use it all the time? Partly because when we use the reflective system, the brain has to work very intensively and a lot of energy is used, which tires the brain out. If we had to go through all the processes involved every time we perform an action, the task would take a very long time to complete. Therefore, the reflective system teaches the automatic to perform tasks with less energy and thought. The automatic processes become habits. What we need to be careful about is not teaching the automatic system bad habits.

The key is to understand how and when to switch on the slow system, and how and when to encourage the fast automatic system to take over. This is not easy, because although the automatic system makes our lives easier in a complex world (all our habitual behaviors like driving, getting to work, doing daily chores like preparing breakfast or a certain household chore, etc).

At the same time, as described earlier, we do not have enough mental power to let the reflective system make all the decisions. We have a limited cognitive bandwidth and we will fail if we ask for more than our concentration can handle. This is why the small details are so important. Having small sub-goals helps us reach our big goals by utilizing the strengths of both systems, and avoiding the pitfalls of each.

. . .

ONE OF THE most important descriptions of how the two systems work in practice is to understand their relationship to 'time'. The automatic system has a strong preference for immediate rewards and prefers to postpone thoughtful, difficult decisions until later. Our reflective system understands that there may be more appropriate decisions to make, but only if the reward is delayed until later ('tomorrow') and that more challenging decisions need to be dealt with today.

EXAMPLE

We tend to succumb to temptations such as cakes, pastries, burgers, crisps, sweets, ice-cream, etc., before merits or benefits that we will receive in the future. Like eating healthy, exercising, clean the house, finishing projects, etc. Because the temptations offer a greater reward in the present.

BEHAVIORAL SCIENTISTS CALL THIS 'PRESENT BIAS' - we prefer rewards today to greater benefits tomorrow, and therefore postpone important decisions and actions, even if we know we shouldn't.

- Reward now (a temptation) instead of gain tomorrow (exercise or eat healthy today)
- We choose cakes and screen time today and put off salad and exercise until tomorrow
- We spend today instead of saving for retirement
- We fail to take care of global problems like climate change because the cost is today and the

benefits of the change can only be seen in the
future

Temptation = reward here and now > 'punishment'
tomorrow (obesity, disease, premature death)

Investment = exercise, healthy eating > gain tomorrow
(healthy, long life, retirement with opportunities)

It is as if we have a *present self* that prefers ice cream, sweets, cakes, beer (temptations) and a *future self*, with a different and healthier frame of reference, such as abstaining from desserts and preferring to drink water. But the problem is, of course, that at some point our future self will be our current self. So if you constantly give in to temptation and put off investing in your health by eating healthy food and exercise, your future self will be penalized. If you're unlucky, that punishment could be a heart attack and instant death.

THE MICROBIOTA - THE BODY'S CONDUCTOR

"I am convinced in the future our medicine cabinets are going to have not just medications like statins for treating us, but also pills that treat and inhibit an enzyme in our microbes and elicit a health benefit in some chronic disease," said Stanley Hazen, MD, PhD, co-section head of Preventive Cardiology & Rehabilitation and director of the Center for Microbiome & Human Health at Cleveland Clinic, Cleveland, Ohio.

Evidence is mounting that the gut microbiome influences just about every major human disease.

By this introduction you probably understand the importance of the gut microbiota and that you do best in taking care of all those billions of microbes if you want to stay healthy.

THE MICROBIOTA CONSISTS of about 100 billion bacteria, viruses, fungi and other microorganisms that live in and on our body. Most live in the gut and mainly in the colon. The total weight of these bacteria (I call the inhabitants of the microbiota bacteria for simplicity and because it consists mainly of bacteria) is about 2 kg and the number of microorganisms in the gut is more than all the cells we have in the body.

IF YOU THINK of the body as a symphony orchestra where our organs are the different sections, then all the musicians involved have to play their instruments in the right place in the piece of music for the orchestra to sound as a unit. To achieve this, the orchestra must be led by a conductor. And the conductor in our body is the microbiota.

THE MICROBIOTA SENDS signals to all our organs through so-called axes (e.g. gut-brain axis, gut-heart axis, gut-skin axis, etc.) These organs can in turn communicate with the microbiota, so if you are stressed or don't sleep well, this can lead to a dysbiosis.

Eating junk food leads to a dysbiosis in the microbiota, which disrupts communication with the organs. When this happens, we may react differently to the dysbiosis, with some suffering from heart problems, others from depression, some from gut diseases, some from overweight and obesity, some from cancer, and some from dementia.

THE MICROBIOTA IS PROBABLY the most important 'organ' in our body and the most important for our health. It also accounts for approximately 80% of our immune system. How badly were you affected by Covid? Those that had a diverse microbiota were less affected and it was probably very few (if any?) who got long-term Covid.

· · ·

WHEN WE EAT JUNK FOOD, stress, sleep poorly, smoke, drink too much alcohol, it leads to a dysbiosis and to a poorer diversity in the microbiota where some bacterial strains can then increase in number and others decrease. The harmony and protection provided by the microbiota is disrupted. This leads to an increase in the number of certain bacteria, which can then become dangerous to us and cause illness. Depending on which bacteria are in majority or in minority, it leads to different types of conditions, such as overweight / obesity, IBS, Inflammatory Bowel Disease, depression, etc. It becomes like a vicious circle when the axes are disrupted.

THE INTERESTING THING is that - and you should take this seriously - when you give the bacteria what they need and want, i.e. fibre, they keep you healthy and give you good health. When you instead eat and drink something that harms the bacteria, such as junk food, sweets, soft drinks and energy drinks, the balance is disturbed and this leads to illness, rapid aging and premature death.

IT'S an interplay where the gut and its inhabitants are the body's most important organs and the engine that drives our well-being. And just like an engine, the microbiota does not want bad fuel because then, just like the engine, it breaks down and, in the worst case, stops permanently.

· · ·

To have a well-functioning microbiota, you should eat fibre. It is the bacteria's food and energy and they literally gorge on fibre. Fibre (dietary fibre - not broken down by gut enzymes but broken down by gut bacteria) is found in carbohydrates such as vegetables, root vegetables, fruits, whole grains, legumes (lentils, beans), whole grain rice. There is fibre that can be digested by bacteria and absorbed into the body and there is fibre that cannot be digested. Both types are important for gut bacteria. Fibre-rich foods also increase satiety and reduce snacking between meals.

Read more under Fibre, Prebiotics, Probiotics and Fermentation.

Western diets have led to the depletion of our microbiota, leading to increasingly poor immune system function and increased morbidity. It is estimated that we have lost 40% of our microbiota compared to the diversity of our ancestral microbiota. Read more under Diets.

Four nutritional factors that gut bacteria crave:

Fibre: When you eat high-fibre foods such as fruit, vegetables, whole grains, nuts and beans, your body cannot process and absorb these fibres as they pass through the upper parts of the gastrointestinal tract. Once they pass through the gut to the lower part (colon), healthy bacteria ferment the food. They produce short-chain fatty acids, which send signals throughout the body, including those related to appetite and satiety.

· · ·

PHENOLS: Phenolic compounds are antioxidants that give plant-based foods their color - when you talk about eating rainbow-colored food, you're talking about phenols. The microbes in your gut also feed on them.

FERMENTED FOODS: You can get health benefits from eating foods that are already fermented - like sauerkraut, kimchi, kefir, yoghurt, miso, tempeh and kombucha. Fermentation can make the phenols in foods more available to the body. In addition, fermented foods add the good bacteria that the gut should consist of, thus increasing the diversity of the microbiota.

FATS: Not so much about feeding the good bacteria in your microbiome. Omega-3 fatty acids, found in oily fish, rapeseed oil, some nuts and other foods, potentially reduce inflammation of the gut lining. In addition, healthy fat sources such as extra virgin olive oil and avocados are full of phenols.

PROGNOSIS ESTIMATE THAT BY 2050, the number of people with chronic diseases will have increased 3 to 4 times. What could happen then is a collapse of the healthcare system, partly due to staff shortages, but also financially, based on healthcare resources and increased prescription of medicines.

YOU SHOULD STRIVE for a diverse microbiome because the

greater the diversity, the better control of body functions you will have.

STUDIES HAVE SHOWN that healthy individuals often have a more diverse gut microbiota. It is also seen in the data that the more beneficial microbes, the more favourably the health outcomes.

One problem for the diversity of the microbiome is that the animals we eat are given antibiotics and the plants are sprayed with pesticides. This tends to limit diversity because you are what you eat and this is also true for the bacteria in the microbiome.

CASES OF COLON cancer are increasingly found in younger people, and it is becoming a problem of epidemic proportions in many countries.

THE MICROBIOTA and food addiction

In a study on both mice and humans, it was found that individuals with food addiction had less of some bacteria and more of others. It was possible to create a food addiction in mice by providing certain bacteria and, conversely, reduce food addiction by providing other types of bacteria.

THE MICROBIOTA CAN INFLUENCE age and heart health

As we age, changes occur in our immune system. Diet, lifestyle and gut function all affect the gut microbiome. This leads to fewer bacterial species, which affects the functioning of the microbiome and thus our overall health and risk of disease.

ONE STUDY LOOKED at 21 markers and divided people into groups. Over 11 years of follow-up, each group's risk of cardiovascular disease was analyzed.

THE OBESE AND high blood sugar groups were 75% and 117% more likely to develop cardiovascular disease, respectively, compared to the 'healthy' groups.

THE GUT MICROBIOME was analyzed to identify bacterial differences between the groups.

THEY IDENTIFIED which bacterial species were present in the microbiome of younger and older people and found 55 bacterial strains that could be linked to age.

ANALYSIS SHOWED that having a microbiome like younger people (microbial age) was associated with a lower risk of cardiovascular disease.

Other studies have shown that dysbiosis can be linked to a range of inflammatory conditions, including inflammatory bowel disease (IBD - Crohn's disease and ulcerative colitis), rheumatoid arthritis and SLE (systemic lupus erythematosus), but also to cardiovascular disease.

· · ·

A **HEALTHY MICROBIOTA** **makes for a strong immune system**

Given that up to 80% of our immune cells (immune system) are found in the gut, any change in bacterial composition also affects our susceptibility to infections and the development of the dangerous inflammation.

THE INTERFACE between the gut bacteria and our immune system is on the surface of the inside of the gut - the layer of cells that forms the gut lining. The intestinal lining is about 400 m^2, equivalent to a very large house. This is a significant surface area that interacts with everything we eat, drink and breathe every day. So it is important that the immune system is always on the alert, processing information and sending the necessary defense elements where they are needed.

THE MICROBIOTA IS like a massive immune processing and distribution centre that protects us from diseases, both locally in the gut and generally in the body, by

- Helping us to break down food into small components
- Promotes gut repair
- Suppresses an overactive inflammatory response
- Prevents pathogens (disease-causing micro-organisms) from sticking to our cells
- Sends T cells to inflamed tissue to protect against infection

- Affects the function of T cells and adapts them to the 'opponent'

ANTIBIOTICS

Antibiotics are drugs that kill bacteria. The first effective anti-infective drug was sulfa, discovered by the German Gerhard Domagk in the 1930s, for which he was awarded the Nobel Prize in Medicine.

An even more widely used antibiotic, which was further developed over the years, was penicillin, discovered by Alexander Fleming in 1928. The difference between sulfa and penicillin is that penicillin kills bacteria by destroying their cell wall. Sulfa inhibits the synthesis of folic acid by bacteria, which prevents them from growing and multiplying. Sulfa is currently used mostly for urinary tract infections.

ANTIBIOTICS KILL ALL BACTERIA, good and bad. In other words, they also destroy the microbiota. This means that when we use antibiotics, we also kill our inherent defenses against infections. This is why we should be very restrictive when using antibiotics.

AN ANECDOTE DESCRIBING ANTIBIOTICS, the microbiota and infection comes from professor of surgery, Stig Bengmark, Lund University Hospital in Sweden.

· · ·

'A junior doctor at the surgical clinic where Stig Bengmark was a professor, had been given the task of analyzing the last 81 major liver operations performed at the hospital. Before presenting the results, he informed Stig that he had both good news and bad news. The bad news was that they had forgotten to give antibiotics to many patients, which, according to the practice at the time, should be given for a week after the operation. This was unacceptable, especially in a university hospital that was supposed to set a good example! However, to Stigs surprise, the young doctor went on to say that 'all the patients who had infections were among those who had received antibiotics - those who had not received antibiotics had not suffered any infection'.

This discovery led Stig to devote much of the rest of his life to studying the microbiota and its importance to our health.

And if you're smart, you'll start today to build up your microbiota and a strong defense against infections and diseases. A strong immune system helps you resist infections and other diseases and reduces the risk of hospitalization. Reports of increased antibiotic resistance should make everyone realize the importance of a strong immune system. And you get that by building a strong microbiota.

And remember - every time you use antibiotics, you destroy your microbiota.

Give your microbiota and your gut bacteria what they want and they will pay you back by giving you many more healthy years of life.

INTERMITTENT FASTING - TIME-RESTRICTED EATING

Time-restricted eating (intermittent fasting) limits when to eat during the day to an 'eating window' of between 8 to 10 hours.

PROVEN BENEFITS of time-restricted eating (TRE) include positive effects on sleep, overweight and obesity, blood sugar regulation, heart function and gut health.

Time-restricted eating may promote longevity and have a positive effect against cancer.

Time-restricted eating involves a regular 24-hour cycle of eating and fasting, with meals strictly limited to the same 8-10 hour window each day. Either you eat breakfast and lunch and nothing more. Or you only eat lunch and dinner. Or breakfast and dinner, but skip lunch.

If you choose either breakfast and lunch or lunch and dinner, you will have two fairly frequent meals and a long fast. This can cause your body to adjust to frequent meals during the day and release insulin in more frequent cycles, which can make you hungry. If you choose to eat breakfast and dinner instead, you'll stretch out your meals and have a more even blood sugar level without insulin secretion. In addition, the gut bacteria get to rest for two longer periods. I myself have chosen to skip lunch. During lunch, I take the opportunity to exercise instead.

Time-restricted eating is a form of intermittent fasting where you can eat for a set period but must refrain from eating for the rest of the day. But you should drink and preferably water.

Researchers believe that intermittent eating improves health and well-being by reinforcing the body's natural daily cycle of rest and activity. But how this works at the molecular level has been unclear.

A study in mice shows that time-restricted eating affects gene activity in 22 different tissues in the body, including the brain, heart, lungs, liver and gut. The findings were published in Cell Metabolism.

Time-restricted eating: what are the benefits?
A review article from 2022 suggests that the health benefits of time-restricted eating include improvements in obesity, diabetes and cardiovascular disease. Fasting can also improve sleep and mental health.

Another study in mice found that time-restricted eating may even have anti-cancer effects.

Crucially, the health benefits of time-restricted eating

compared to eating at any time during the day appear to apply regardless of total calories or type of food consumed.

Time-restricted eating has been shown to be beneficial for the body's circadian rhythm (in all tissues studied), which includes our natural cycles of rest and activity.

Time-restricted eating reduced the activity of genes involved in inflammation and increased the activity of genes involved in autophagy - the disposal and recycling of old and damaged cell parts.

INCREASED AUTOPHAGY, but only during the period of fasting, is known to improve health by preventing and managing age-related diseases.

Increased inflammation and decreased autophagy are well-known hallmarks of biological aging.

The microbiome is working full-time so when you fast or eat less, you rest the microbiome so that energy can be replenished, just like when you sleep. This is definitely one of the theories of why you improve the diversity of the microbiome with time-restricted eating.

A DANGER for many people is that when you've been fasting for 12 to 16 hours, you tend eat too much when you do eat again. So it's important to be vigilant and only eat a predetermined amount of food.

Although shift work is unavoidable for many people, it is associated with an increased risk of obesity, diabetes, heart disease and cancer as a result of disruptions to the body's circadian rhythm.

In theory, time-restricted eating can help restore these

rhythms and boost the health and well-being of shift workers.

One study found that time-restricted eating improved the physical and mental health of firefighters working regular 24-hour shifts.

THERE ARE many studies underway to find out the benefits of time-restricted eating, including more than 150 studies examining the effects on:

- obesity
- type 2 diabetes
- hypertension
- high cholesterol
- heart disease
- cancer

COMMENTS BY RESEARCHERS on time-restricted eating:

'Time-restricted eating can reduce hunger as a result of lower insulin response and thus lead to weight loss. I have found intermittent fasting to be an extremely effective tool for my patients who need to lose weight, and a big plus is that it discourages rushed snacking, which is a problem for many. Of course, what is eaten needs to be considered, especially by those who have diabetes.'

Kimberly Gomer, RD, Dietitian at Body Beautiful Miami Florida, USA

· · ·

'TIME-RESTRICTED eating is known to improve microbiota, liver health, blood sugar regulation, muscle function (increased endurance capacity), sleep quality, cognitive function and resistance to infectious disease'.

Professor Satchidananda Panda, Ph.D., Salk Institute for Biological Studies in La Jolla, California, USA

WHAT, HOW, HOW MUCH AND WHEN TO EAT

Calorie is a unit of energy and a measure of the energy content of food, i.e. the energy we need to carry out our daily activities. Too much energy leads to weight gain and too little leads to weight loss. Some foods contain many calories per gram and others fewer.

How much energy you need depends mainly on three things:

1. How much energy your body spends at rest
2. How much energy is needed to break down and absorb the food you eat
3. How physical active you are

The nutrients that provide energy are protein, carbohydrates, fat, alcohol and dietary fibre.

· · ·

THE AMOUNT of calories (kcal) in 1 gram is:
protein - 4 kcal
carbohydrates - 4 kcal
fat - 9 kcal
alcohol - 7 kcal
dietary fibre 2 kcal

WHEN IT COMES to alcohol as an energy source, several factors come into play.

You want to lose weight and you have a dinner and drink alcohol. The calories from the food will not be burnt until the alcohol has been burnt and eliminated. Because alcohol is toxic to the body, the liver works to get rid of it first. This in turn means that fat burning is reduced and fat is stored in your body. Alcohol also leads to increased hunger, so you need to be vigilant. This may not always be easy if you've been to a party and pass a fast food restaurant on your way home.

WITH THIS GUIDE, we identify the traps and create strategies on how to avoid them. Just knowing what can happen after a night of partying might make you either take a different route home and avoid the fast food, or bring a banana, some nuts or something else healthy to eat. But only a little, because all calories count and, as mentioned above, alcohol is burned first and other calories risk being stored as fat.

HOW MUCH ENERGY do we need?

The amount of energy (calorie) we need depends on our gender and how much physical activity we engage in.

Depending on activity - Low activity (LA) Medium activity (MA) High activity (HA)

Women (calorie)

18 - 24 yrs 2000 (LA) 2200 (MA) 2500 (HA)

25 - 50 yrs 1900 (LA) 2200 (MA) 2400 (HA)

51 >70 yrs 1700 (LA) 2000 (MA) 2200 (HA)

MEN (CALORIE)

8 - 24 yrs 2500 (LA) 2800 (MA) 3200 (HA)

25 - 50 yrs 2400 (LA) 2700 (MA) 3000 (HA)

51 - 70 yrs 2200 (LA) 2500 (MA) 2800 (HA)

>70 yrs 2100 (LA) 2400 (MA) 2700 (HA)

NOW THAT YOU know your needs based on age and physical activity, it's time to calculate how much you eat and drink. To really know where you stand, you need to be honest with yourself. Everything you put in your mouth must be taken into account. To find out more about how to calculate your intake, see the chapter on Nutrient content.

How should the energy percentage be distributed?

According to the new Nordic Nutrition Recommendations, the distribution between the energy-giving nutrients protein, fat and carbohydrates should be

Protein 10-20%

Fat 25-40%

Carbohydrates 45-60%

. . .

SOURCE: Swedish National Food Agency

EAT SLOWLY

Meals eaten quickly, energy dense food and extra tasty food are 3 factors that increase the risk of gaining weight.

The main cause of obesity is prolonged imbalance in energy intake - consuming more calories than the body makes use of.

It usually takes about 20 minutes for the satiety signals to reach your brain. If you then eat a large meal in just 10 minutes, it will take a while for the brain to register the satiety signals and the risk of overeating increases. When we eat foods that are unprocessed (fruit, vegetables, legumes, whole grains, etc.), we eat fewer calories, more dietary fibre and those foods are less calorific. The more calories, the more energy-dense the food.

EXAMPLE OF CALORIE content (calories per 100 grams - 3,5 Oz)

- Potatoes 79
- French fries 307
- Potato chips 495

Note what happens to the potato when it is processed. French fries and potato chips do not contain any direct nutrients and the process they undergo leads is bad for the microbiota.

- Beef mince 205
- Beef 106
- Broccoli 35
- Cauliflower 24
- Cucumber 13

A simple comparison - 1 kg (2,2 lb) of cauliflower contains about as many calories as 100 grams of minced beef. And a lot more fibre.

Grilled meat and DNA damage

High temperature cooking can damage the DNA of food. Scientists believe that damaged DNA can be absorbed during digestion, and then make its way into the DNA of the person eating it.

A study from June 2023 indicates that consuming damaged food DNA may pose a genetic risk to the person consuming it.

Beef mince, pork mince and sliced potatoes were cooked by either boiling the food for 15 minutes at 100 degrees Celsius or roasting it in an oven at 220 degrees Celsius for 20 minutes.

It was found that all three foods showed DNA damage both when cooked and roasted. Food cooked at higher temperatures showed increased DNA damage.

Potatoes showed less DNA damage than meat. This may be because plants contain less DNA per weight than animals.

The types of DNA damage caused by the food were genotoxic, which means that it can impair the function of genes and stimulate gene mutations that can cause cancer.

This may be one reason why we pass on damaged genes that can lead to disease in children and adolescents.

MEAL LENGTH AFFECTS whether children eat fruit and vegetables

Getting children to eat vegetables can be difficult. In most cases, it is a matter of mum and dad having to eat fruit and vegetables for their children to do so. Children imitate their parents. Forcing children to eat what their parents do not eat will not succeed. You can't put the onus on schools to get children to eat fruit and vegetables. That responsibility should be yours as a parent.

One study found that children aged 6 to 11 ate significantly more fruit and vegetables when family meals lasted about 10 minutes longer than usual.

Not stressing at mealtimes can have a positive effect on children's desire to eat fruit and vegetables.

DON'T EAT LATE at night

You are what you eat, as the saying goes. But a growing body of evidence suggests that it's not just what and how much you eat that affects your health, but when and how fast you eat also matters. Research now suggests that these two factors can increase the risk of gastrointestinal problems, obesity and type 2 diabetes.

So, ideally, eat your last meal of the day at 6 p.m. Eating earlier than this increases the risk of feeling full and craving something in the evening that you wouldn't have eaten if you were full.

6

FOODS TO AVOID

Most people know that a big cheeseburger with fries is unhealthy. And that pizza can be. And that fried chicken is. And cake and other pastries. And ice cream and sweets. Or do you know that? Maybe you just don't care? Life should be good.

But what about the knowledge of which products harm us and how, and in the long term cause illness and premature death? Do you want to know? Maybe not, but if you want to be healthy and live long, you have no choice.

Being a consumer is not easy. And that's one of the reasons for this guide. To make it easy to eat and drink right. And to recognise and navigate past other dangers that lurk in everyday life.

THE NOTION that 'eating it once in a while can't be that bad' is certainly true. But 'once in a while' has a tendency to become quite frequent. For example, Saturday candy are certainly 'once in a while' for some. But 'Saturdays' happen every week, so it hardly becomes 'once in a while'. Then it is perhaps not so unusual to buy Saturday candy on Friday and thus extend Saturday. And then continue over to Sunday. In other words, weekend candy.

THIS GUIDE IS MEANT to give you a better understanding of the consequences of how you live your life so that you can make better decisions about whether you think it's worth changing your lifestyle or whether you want to take a chance and continue eating unhealthy things.

If you are currently eating healthy, this will confirm that you are already making the right decisions. If you think you're eating healthy, you may find that you're actually not and you can correct unhealthy details. In the end, it is you who decides how you want to live your life.

Whatever we do in life, whatever decisions we make, there will always be a consequence. If you want your taste buds to decide what to eat, there will be consequences to that decision.

In a similar way to continuing to smoke. Everyone knows that smoking causes disease and shortens lives.

So every decision you make leads to a consequence!

ULTRA-PROCESSED foods are products that are altered from their origin beyond recognition. A rule of thumb is that when you look at the list of ingredients of products and they contain more than 5 ingredients, and often with a high content of sugar, salt, saturated fat, as well as substances such as emulsifiers, thickeners, preservatives, then they are ultra-processed products.

Examples include sausages, charcuterie (salami, spicy sausages, liver pate, etc.), frozen pizzas, cakes ('biscuits'), nuggets, candy, ice cream, soft drinks (both sugar-sweetened and artificially sweetened), energy drinks, etc.

ALL of these products are designed to make you addicted to them and to make it difficult to stop eating and drinking them. The more you eat and drink these ultra-processed products, the more you will crave them.

STUDIES HAVE SHOWN why it is so difficult to give up ultra-processed products. These foods seem to be able to cause an 'ultra-processed food addiction', an addiction fully comparable to addictive stimulants like tobacco and alcohol.

SOME FOODS ARE MORE likely to cause an addiction than others. In one study, participants mentioned chocolate, pizza, French fries, potato chips and soft drinks as some of the most addictive foods. These foods are all high in refined carbohydrates, fat or salt and at much higher levels than those found in natural foods (e.g. fruit, vegetables, beans).

It was found that around 14% of adults and 12% of children showed significant signs of being dependent on these foods. Addiction rates among adults are similar to those for legal substances such as alcohol and tobacco. Behaviors and brain mechanisms involved in the development of addictive disorders, such as craving and impulsivity, were also seen in the consumption of ultra-processed products.

Many ultra-processed products have the same effect on our brain as nicotine. People who always have a Coca Cola in their hand are likely to be ultra-processed dependent. Whether it is a regular coke or a diet coke (see below on artificial sweeteners). The same goes for those who drink energy drinks. Consumers say it's good, but the truth is that they are ultra-processed dependent.

ULTRA-PROCESSED products cause a dysbiosis in the microbiota resulting in a less resilient intestinal mucosa. This leads to the intestinal mucosa becoming less resistant and leaking contents from the gut into their bloodstream, that a healthy intestinal mucosa resists. This is known as a leaky gut.

Ultra-processed products cause inflammatory processes in the body. Inflammation increases the risk of heart disease, mental health problems, cancer, inflammatory bowel disease, dementia, etc.

Also avoid vegan products that are ultra-processed. These contain the same unhealthy substances. Always read the product's ingredient list.

Also avoid products that contain emulsifiers (see the chapter on Food additives). Emulsifiers have been linked to an increased risk of cardiovascular disease and various types of cancer. Also avoid products that contain thickeners, colorings, etc. These additives are more the rule than the exception in ultra-processed products.

Avoid artificial sweeteners. There are increasing reports that sweeteners such as xylitol, aspartame, sucralose, erythritol, etc. increase the risk of cardiovascular disease. Sweeteners have also been found to increase hunger, which can lead to weight gain. Switching from sugar-sweetened food or drinks to low-calorie products with artificial sweeteners is not a solution if you want to lose weight.

Sweeteners also cause a dysbiosis in the microbiota. The fact that a product contains an artificial substance signals that it is 'unnatural'. So avoid it.

. . .

SATURATED FAT (READ MORE UNDER 'FATS')

If you want to avoid gaining weight or if you want to lose weight, avoid foods high in saturated fat.

The recommendation from the world's experts is to reduce the amount of saturated fat as it increases the risk of obesity and cardiovascular disease.

IN THE SWEDISH study known as the 'Muffin Study', participants were given muffins containing either saturated fat or polyunsaturated fat. Both groups gained weight, but those who ate saturated fat developed an accumulation of fat around the intestines, i.e. visceral fat. Abdominal obesity is known to be particularly dangerous for developing diseases such as type 2 diabetes and cardiovascular disease.

A LOT of saturated fat is found in cheese, both hard and soft. The fat content is usually expressed as a percentage, for example '28% mature cheese'. 28% means that almost a third of the cheese consists of fat, 28 grams out of 100 grams. Of this, about 2/3 is saturated fat.

COLD CUTS SUCH AS SAUSAGES, bacon, cassoulet, smoked ham, salami, liver pate and black pudding are also high in saturated fat. If you want to continue eating meat while losing weight and staying healthy, you should eliminate cold cuts from your diet in the first place, as they contain salt, nitrites, nitrates and other additives that are bad for your health.

. . .

Reduce the amount of meat you eat if you eat a lot, as the risk of developing disease is directly related to the amount you consume, according to most studies.

Vegan products can also be high in saturated fat and additives such as thickeners, colorings, flavor enhancers, emulsifiers, salt, etc.

Many vegan products contain coconut oil as a binding agent and coconut oil contains over 90% saturated fat. The earlier coconut oil is mentioned in the list of ingredients, the more of it there is. When you look at the nutrition labelling, you will see that the percentage of saturated fat is high.

Do you want to eat meat and fish? The recommendations from health organizations are to eat meat in moderation and to eat only meat from pastured (or wild) animals and sea-caught fish. Industrial meat and farmed fish contain, among other things, concentrated feed and medicines. If you eat these animals you will obviously ingest these products too. Organic products, both animal and plant-based, are preferable if you want to avoid ingesting chemicals.

In September 2024, it was reported that the salmon lice rate in farmed salmon in northern Norway is at a record high. Usually 0.5 adult lice per fish are accepted. Now, 4 lice per fish have been found, which is 8 times higher than the permitted limit.

. . .

WE MUST REALIZE that the only thing the food industry and food chains are striving for is to make more money. On us as consumers.

To avoid being fooled by their tricks, we need to be smarter than them and resist when they market their temptations in different ways. Try to be observant of how tempting their adverts are.

IN GROCERY STORES, unhealthy junk products with high margins, such as soft drinks, sweets, crisps, etc. are placed in strategic locations where we and our children pass by. The food chains have no objective to promote our health. They ONLY want our money.

BUT WHAT IF you eat sea-caught fish?

Fish tend to accumulate heavy metals and chemicals. The fatter the fish, the higher the levels. Authorities warn against eating lake fish or too much fish from the Baltic Sea. Pregnant women in particular are advised not to eat these fish.

When it comes to fish caught in our western seas, you risk ingesting chemicals, heavy metals and microplastics.

THERE ARE five eddies in our oceans: two in the Atlantic, two in the Pacific and one in the Indian Ocean. Here, huge accumulations of debris form in the so-called *ocean gyres*. The most famous is *the Great Pacific Garbage Patch*.

Lots of plastic debris accumulates in the gyres and the plastic is mostly made up of very small plastic fragments that are not visible from the surface but are present throughout the water mass right down to the bottom.

ONE REASON why there is so much plastic in the oceans is because fishing gear has been left behind or has worn out. It is estimated that around 50% of the plastic in the oceans comes from fishing gear. We have been told that plastic straws are responsible for a significant amount of marine litter and have therefore been banned, accounting for only about 0.03% of all plastic.

LARGE PLASTIC PRODUCTS in the oceans gradually break down into microplastics that are so small they are invisible. The microplastics bind to algae and plankton, which are eaten by smaller fish and shellfish, which in turn are eaten by larger fish, which are eaten by even larger fish, which are eaten by humans. Microplastics are absorbed into the bloodstream via the gut and end up in different parts of the body.

We also breathe in microplastics, so it can be difficult to completely prevent them from entering our bodies. However, if we choose not to eat fish, we are at least avoiding a large amount of plastic.

ANOTHER FACTOR that is rarely mentioned is that when fish swim from deep water to the surface, they create a downward vortex in the water that pulls down the carbon dioxide that the oceans collect from the atmosphere, and stores it deep down on the seabed. And the oceans' capacity to sequester carbon dioxide is far greater than the rainforest. By trawling all the fish, including by-catch (which is enormous), the Earth is losing this carbon sequestration resource.

Speaking of the enormous amount of by-catch that is caught in trawling and thrown back into the sea. This by-catch leads to an advanced disruption of the marine ecosystem.

So WHY IS nothing being done about overfishing?

Because large amounts of money are involved.

Because it is difficult to control fishing quotas because illegal fishing is so advanced.

Because the fishing lobby is very strong.

Because many people depend on the fishing industry.

Because politicians are politicians and mainly prioritize their own position and power.

BUT YOU CAN CHOOSE whether to support your children's future by opting out of fish on your plate.

INFLAMMATORY AND ANTI-INFLAMMATORY FOODS

I nflammatory diet

Inflammation plays an important role in the onset of diseases. Foods are known to cause inflammation in the body and these foods are called pro-inflammatory foods.

EXPERTS RECOMMEND AVOIDING the following foods that causes inflammation:

- Red meat such as steak, burgers, offal
- Processed meat such as bacon and sausages
- Industrial baked goods like cakes, pies and brownies
- Bread and pasta made with white flour
- Deep-fried products such as French fries, fried chicken and doughnuts
- Foods high in added sugar such as sweets and ice cream
- Chips, cheesecake, etc.

- Sugar-sweetened drinks such as soft drinks and sports energy drinks
- Dairy products (the dairy industry believes that it does not)
- Food additives such as thickeners, emulsifiers, stabilisers, colorings
- Trans fats found in margarine, microwave popcorn, biscuits

Systemic inflammation can become chronic and persist for months or even years.

CHRONIC, systemic inflammation is the cause of diseases such as:

- Obesity
- Metabolic syndrome
- Type 2 diabetes
- Heart disease
- Stroke
- Inflammatory bowel disease, including Crohn's disease and ulcerative colitis
- Some forms of cancer
- Arthritis
- Alzheimer's disease

IN SIMPLE TERMS, the process works as follows:
You eat and drink products that cause a dysbiosis in the microbiota. This leads to a deterioration in the protective function of the intestinal mucosa and allows 'dangerous'

substances from the food to pass through. This triggers a variety of processes that lead to low-grade inflammation, including damage to the walls of the heart's blood vessels, allowing cholesterol to build up and clog the vessels. Inflammation also damages cells in the body, which in turn causes disease.

It's not an overnight process, it goes on for years. You can stop inflammation by avoiding unhealthy foods and drinks and adding more healthy ingredients into your diet.

Read more under 'Microbiota'.

LIKE SO MANY other unhealthy factors in our lives, inflammation increases with the amount of products you eat. So it's a question of dose. But it also depends on individual sensitivity. Some people's bodies can take more of a beating. Everyone gets sick sooner or later if they eat a lot of unhealthy food, so whether that happens at 50, 60 or 70 will become apparent.

IN ADDITION to cutting down on pro-inflammatory foods, you can increase your consumption of anti-inflammatory foods.

ANTI-INFLAMMATORY DIET

Anti-inflammatory diets are diets that counteract or reduce inflammation in the body. There is no single superfood that works directly. But you can reduce inflammation over time by eating a variety of nutritious foods daily.

· · ·

An anti-inflammatory diet should include these foods:

- tomatoes
- olive oil
- green leafy vegetables, such as spinach, kale, rocket
- fermented vegetables, kimchi
- beans, lentils (legumes)
- nuts such as walnuts and pecans
- dark yellow vegetables such as carrots, pumpkin, sweet potato
- soya, cabbage, onion, garlic, leek, broccoli, quinoa
- whole grains
- oily fish such as salmon (avoid farmed salmon), mackerel, tuna and sardines
- fruit and berries such as strawberries, blueberries, cherries and oranges
- tea, coffee

Benefits of anti-inflammatory diets

Drinks and foods that reduce inflammation also lead to a lower risk of chronic diseases. Fruits and vegetables such as blueberries, apples and leafy greens that are high in natural antioxidants and polyphenols (protective compounds) have been found to be particularly beneficial.

Studies have also shown that nuts reduce

inflammation and thus the risk of cardiovascular disease and diabetes.

Coffee, which contains polyphenols and other anti-inflammatory compounds, may also protect against inflammation. But too much coffee can be unhealthy.

BIOMARKERS:

A biomarker is a biological molecule found in blood, other body fluids or tissues that indicates whether everything is working properly or whether there is an abnormal process such as a disease.

COMMON BIOMARKERS USED in studies to identify inflammation in the body are **CRP (C-reactive protein), Interleukin 6 and TNFα-R2.**

CRP IS ALSO USED as a 'rapid infectious disease marker' when healthcare professionals check for infection. However, now we are looking for an inflammation and not an infection. The difference between infection and inflammation is that an infection is caused by a virus, a bacterium or a fungus and an inflammation is not. It can be caused by other triggers.

Inflammation means that the body's immune system has reacted to an injury or attack. An infection almost always leads to an inflammation. Both conditions activate the body's immune system.

The biomarker CRP is used in both infection and inflammation, but in different ways and with different sensitivities.

. . .

To CHECK if you have a low-grade systemic inflammation in your body, a blood test called **hs-CRP** (high-sensitivity CRP), is used.

THE NORMAL VALUE for CRP when looking for an infection is <3 (less than 3), but this value is far too high if you want to know if you have a low-grade inflammation.

Your hs-CRP should be as close to 0 (zero) as possible to indicate that you do not have an inflammation.

IF YOU ASK your doctor to check for inflammation - be firm that you should have a referral for hs-CRP.

IT IS VERY important to know your health status. Therefore, the healthcare system examines us with various blood tests, blood pressure, ECG, etc. partly to have baseline values and partly to follow up treatments and advice and see if we get healthier, sicker or an unchanged health status. It is always you who decides what you want the outcome of your treatment to be.

SOMETIMES IT CAN BE difficult to get a test for hs-CRP and this is probably due to both cost and lack of knowledge.

However, if you take this new information with you and argue convincingly with your doctor, you will improve your chances of getting the blood test.

You can also buy the test from a private provider.

8

DIETS - THREE GOOD ONES AND ONE BAD (BUT COMMON) ONE

This chapter describes 3 healthy diets and a less healthy one. The healthy diets are the Mediterranean diet, the DASH diet and the plant-based diet and the unhealthy one is the Western diet.

THE UNHEALTHY DIET, the so-called Western diet, is actually the one that many of us eat. It is the diet that has been found to be responsible for the majority of our lifestyle diseases. It is a major contributor to overweight, obesity, cardiovascular disease, cancer, dementia, depression, etc.

MANY PEOPLE USE the term lifestyle diseases without realizing that these diseases are caused by the way we live. Diet is a strong contributing factor to the onset of these diseases.

•   •   •

The German Hausmannskost means 'simple diet'. And this type of food is probably common in most western countries, but with local ingredients.

And if we call it hausmannskost, it must be good and healthy food, right? Unfortunately, far from all home-cooked meals are. Many dishes include processed and ultra-processed products such as sausages, bacon, hamburgers etc. And home-cooked dishes such as mashed potatoes with pork, white rice with stew, pasta with meat sauce etc. can be high in saturated fat, high in cholesterol, carbohydrates, salt and low in fibre.

If you eat meat, it is recommended that you chose meat from grazing cows and not from the meat industry, whether domestic or foreign. The same goes for pork, chicken and fish (and avoid farmed salmon).

The Nordic Nutrition Recommendations says no more than 350 grams meat per week. Add plenty of vegetables to your diet.

Mediterranean diet

The Mediterranean diet is the most studied and scientifically documented diet and is considered the diet that best prevents cardiovascular disease. In May 2024, a review of studies was published which concluded that only the Mediterranean diet could prevent cardiovascular disease and cardiac death.

'Mediterranean diet' is a generic term based on the traditional eating habits of countries bordering the Mediterranean Sea. There is no generalised Mediterranean diet. At least 16 countries border the Mediterranean. Diets vary between these countries and also between regions within each country due to differences in culture, ethnicity, religion, economy, geography and agricultural production. However, there are some common denominators.

A MEDITERRANEAN DIET USUALLY INCLUDES:

- Lots of vegetables, fruit, beans, lentils and nuts
- Lots of whole grains, such as whole grain bread and brown or black rice
- Lots of extra virgin olive oil (EVOO) which is a source of healthy fat
- Small to moderate amounts of fish, especially fish rich in omega-3 fatty acids
- Small to moderate amounts of natural cheese, yoghurt and eggs
- Little or no red meat, choose poultry, fish or beans instead of red meat

Fish and poultry are more common than red meat in this diet. It also focuses on minimally processed, plant-based foods and recommends fresh and natural products. Wine can be consumed in small to moderate amounts, usually accompanied by meals. Fruit is a common dessert instead of sweets.

THE MEDITERRANEAN DIET has many benefits, including:

- Reducing the risk of cardiovascular disease, including heart attack and stroke
- Contributes to a healthy body weight

- Contributes to healthy blood sugar levels, blood pressure and cholesterol.
- Reduces the risk of metabolic syndrome - metabolic syndrome is an umbrella term for a number of factors that increase the risk of lifestyle diseases such as cardiovascular disease, type 2 diabetes and also some common cancers such as prostate, bowel and breast cancer. More recently, it has also been suggested that metabolic syndrome may play a significant role in the development of certain types of dementia. Recent studies also show that people with metabolic syndrome are five times more likely to have a heart attack
- Contributes to a healthy balance of the microbiota
- Reduces the risk of certain types of cancer
- Slows the decline in brain function as you age
- Helps you live longer

THE MEDITERRANEAN DIET has these benefits because it:

- Limits the intake of saturated and trans fats. Eating too much saturated fat can raise your LDL (bad) cholesterol. High LDL increases the risk of plaque build-up in your arteries (atherosclerosis). Trans fats have no health benefits. Both of these 'unhealthy fats' can cause inflammation in your body.
- Favor healthy unsaturated fats, including omega-3 fatty acids. Unsaturated fats promote

healthy cholesterol levels, support brain health and fight inflammation. In addition, a diet high in unsaturated fats and low in saturated fats promotes healthy blood sugar levels.

- Limiting salt (sodium) intake. Eating foods high in sodium can raise your blood pressure, putting you at higher risk of heart attack or stroke.
- Limit your intake of refined carbohydrates, including sugar. Foods high in refined carbohydrates cause your blood sugar to rise quickly. Refined carbohydrates also give you excess calories that have no nutritional benefits. These foods also often lack fibre.
- Foods high in fibre and antioxidants. These nutrients help reduce inflammation in the body. Fibre also stimulates better bowel movements and less risk of constipation. Fibre also helps maintain healthy blood sugar levels. Antioxidants protect you against cancer by eliminating free radicals.

The Mediterranean diet contains many different nutrients that work together in the body for better health. There is no single food or ingredient that is solely responsible for the benefits of the Mediterranean diet. It is healthy because of the combination of nutrients included.

IMAGINE A CHOIR OF SINGERS. One voice may be able to carry part of the song, but you need all voices to achieve the full effect. In the same way, the Mediterranean diet works by providing you with a perfect blend of nutrients that together build up your health.

. . .

DASH-diet

DASH stands for 'Dietary Approaches to Stop Hypertension' and is a result of American research on hypertension.

The DASH diet is a healthy diet designed to prevent or treat high blood pressure. The diet can also help lower low-density lipoprotein (LDL) cholesterol, which is a risk marker for cardiovascular disease.

High blood pressure and high LDL cholesterol are two serious risk factors for heart disease and stroke.

Foods recommended in the DASH diet are rich in the minerals potassium, calcium and magnesium while limiting intake of foods high in salt (sodium), added sugars and saturated fats, such as meat and dairy products.

The DASH diet includes vegetables, fruit, whole grains, beans, nuts, low-fat dairy products, fish, chicken.

Plant-based diet

A plant-based diet aims to eliminate all animal products, such as meat, poultry, fish, eggs, dairy products. Everything you eat comes from plants such as whole grains, fruits, vegetables, legumes, lentils, nuts and seeds.

A plant-based diet has significant health benefits as long as you do it the right way.

No matter when you start, a plant-based diet will prevent many diseases and make you feel better.

. . .

IF FOLLOWED CORRECTLY, a plant-based diet limits the intake of added sugars, processed foods, additives and instead recommends whole food, fresh and nutritious foods. It maximizes nutrient intake and eliminates foods that are unhealthy.

A plant-based diet is low in saturated fat, free of cholesterol and rich in fibre, vitamins, minerals and antioxidants.

RESEARCH ALSO SHOWS that a plant-based diet reduces the risk of:

- Heart disease
- Hypertension (high blood pressure)
- Diabetes
- Gastrointestinal diseases
- Colon cancer
- Breast cancer
- Obesity

STUDIES ALSO SHOW that a plant-based diet can contribute to weight loss and lower bad LDL cholesterol.

A plant-based diet is often expressed as a vegan diet, so it's easy to confuse the two.

But there is an important difference. Both diets involves only to eat foods from the plants.

Veganism, on the other hand, is more than just about the diet - it's a way of life. Most vegans avoid using, consuming or exploiting animals. For example, they may choose not to buy or use products made from or tested on animals.

A plant-based eating pattern focuses on whole and mostly fresh foods, so it avoids packaged and processed products. A vegan may consume frozen meat options or vegan snacks and desserts, while a person following a plant-based diet will instead eat protein in the form of legumes, soybean, nuts and a dessert with fruit instead of processed vegan ice cream.

Suggestions on how to start eating a plant-based diet

Keep it simple! Start by removing one animal product at a time and replace it with a plant-based one.

For example, you can first replace milk and dairy products with soya, oat, almond alternatives. Use plant-based alternatives to yoghurt and kefir, and soy or oat drinks in your coffee. But be aware of additives. Plant-based milk stored on a room tempered shelf in the food store does contain additives.

Then replace chicken, turkey, beef, pork, veal, lamb and fish with plant proteins.

Top up with legumes, beans, nuts, seeds and vegan protein alternatives such as homemade tofu veggie burgers, nutritional yeast and tempeh. Note that they should not contain unhealthy additives such as emulsifiers, thickeners, preservatives, etc.

Make sure to include all five food groups at every meal - plant protein, fruit, vegetables, plant-based fat (extra virgin olive oil) and whole grains.

Suggestions:

· · ·

BREAKFAST: muesli with oats, chopped nuts, fresh berries, fruit and sunflower and pumpkin seeds.

LUNCH: Veggie burrito with a whole grain tortilla, beans, mixed vegetables, tomatoes, peppers, onions and nutritional yeast. Pair with corn tortilla chips and fresh salsa or guacamole.

DINNER: Scrambled tofu with brown or black rice and various vegetables sautéed in olive oil.

You **WANT** your diet to contain enough protein to maintain muscle mass, strong bones and healthy skin. The following foods are packed with protein:

- Beans, lentils and peas
- Quinoa
- Soy products such as tempeh, tofu, soybeans
- Nuts and seeds

You **ALSO NEED** to get enough calcium and vitamin D in your diet for bone building.

- Drink a milk alternative such as soya, almond, oat milk, which contains both calcium and vitamin D.

- Eat dark leafy vegetables, green salad and beans.
- Eat mushrooms and fortified cereals that contain vitamin D. If you do not consume fortified foods on a consistent basis, you need to take a vitamin D supplement. Sunlight is the natural source of vitamin D.

You ALSO NEED enough zinc in your diet to build a healthy immune system, enough iron to maintain energy and immunity, and enough vitamin B12 to produce red blood cells and prevent anaemia.

You GET THIS IF YOU:

Eat whole grains, beans, tofu and fortified cereals with zinc and iron.

Eat nutritional yeast and soya products to get vitamin B12. You should take vitamin B12 supplements.

WESTERN diet

The Western diet is a diet generally characterised by a high intake of pre-packaged foods, refined grains, red meat, processed meat, high-sugar drinks, sweets and crisps, fried foods, industrially produced animal products, butter and other high-fat dairy products, eggs, potatoes, maize (and high-fructose corn syrup) and a low intake of fruit, vegetables, whole grains, pasture-raised animal products, fish, nuts and seeds.

· · ·

COMPARED to the Mediterranean diet and similar healthy diets that are higher in fruits, vegetables, whole grains and moderate intake of fish and chicken, the Western diet is associated with higher risks of cardiovascular disease and obesity.

FOODS INCLUDED in this diet have been so heavily processed that it has fundamentally altered 7 nutritional characteristics:

- glycaemic load
- composition of fatty acids
- macronutrient composition (protein, fat, carbohydrates)
- micronutrient density (vitamins and minerals), acid-base balance
- sodium-potassium ratio and fibre content.

IMPORTANT

The Western diet has a negative impact on metabolism (weight gain), increases inflammation (which causes diseases) and decreases the absorption of antioxidants (which protect us from disease), leads to a dysbiosis in the gut microbiota (which protects us from many diseases and is responsible for about 80% of our immune system) and has a negative effect on cardiovascular health, mental health, cancer, etc.

The Western diet is the main reason for the rapid development of the current obesity epidemic.

9

FIBRES

F ibre is food for our gut bacteria. The billions of bacteria, viruses and fungi that live in the gut and especially in the colon are called the microbiota.

FROM FIBRE, the bacteria produce beneficial substances that strengthen the intestinal mucosa so that it can resist toxins that we ingest (it's called intestinal or gut leakage, and means that the intestinal mucosa lets through substances that a healthy intestinal mucosa would never do), provide fuel for the intestinal bacteria that account for about 80% of our immune system and thus protect against various diseases. We used to eat about 150 grams of plant fibre a day, but we are far from that amount today. Back then, we also had more than twice as rich a microbiota (diversity), both in terms of the total number of bacteria and the number of species (bacteria strains). People in general, especially those suffering from increased inflammation in the body such as obese people, have a much lower diversity in their microbiota, and have thus lost the bacteria that break down fibre, because they have not 'fed' these bacteria. The lost bacteria include some lactobacilli.

UNRIPE FRUITS and vegetables are very rich in both fibre and antioxidants.

When plant fibres ripen, they are converted into sugar, for example, unripe bananas are extremely rich in fibre, especially pectin, but when the banana ripens, it is converted into sugar and calories. So if you want a banana with fibre, buy green bananas, the ones that are hard to peel, hard and tough when you eat them. You can easily slice the banana and freeze it to use in smoothies, for example. You can do the same with unripe avocados or buy frozen avocados.

FOUR FIBRES

FOUR FIBRES with beneficial health effects are pectin, inulin, beta-glucans and resistant starch.

PECTIN

100% of the pectin we eat reaches the colon and the microbiota. Pectin is abundant in citrus fruits, especially in grapefruit (if you are taking medicine, read the package leaflet and find out if your medicine is affected by grapefruit - many medicines do not work with grapefruit), apples (mostly in the peel), unripe bananas, apricots, blackberries, raspberries, strawberries, peaches, etc.

Pectin has a unique ability to reduce *metabolic*

syndrome and lower levels of LDL cholesterol (the bad cholesterol) in the blood, known as a risk factor for cardiovascular disease. Pectin can also effectively inhibit diarrhoea. The more fruits and berries containing pectin you eat daily, the better effect you will get from it.

INULIN

Inulin is the fibre most studied for its health effects. Inulin belongs to a group of carbohydrates called fructans, and they are abundant in the herb chicory (cultivated varieties are frisée lettuce and rose salad), Jerusalem artichoke, garlic, leek and common onion. Dandelion leaves are also rich in inulin and so are bananas, albeit only in small amounts.

Unfortunately, large parts of the population have lost the gut bacteria that break down these fibres and eating more than 2-3 grams of inulin a day can cause intestinal problems such as gas, bloating, nausea, abdominal cramps, diarrhoea or constipation.

Inulin has been shown to help increase insulin sensitivity, reduce metabolic syndrome and prevent the development of type 2 diabetes.

BETA-GLUCANS

Beta-glucans are mainly found in the cereals oats and barley, in various mushrooms such as shiitake, maitake, reishi, shimeji and in dates. Beta-glucans have been shown in studies to lower levels of harmful LDL cholesterol, and in the United States, beta-glucans are allowed to be marketed as a product with a heart-protective effect.

Consuming 3 grams (0,1 oz) of beta-glucan from oats

has been shown to lower cholesterol levels. In addition to heart-protective effects, studies have also shown that beta-glucans can:

- protect against antibiotic-resistant strains
- protect against cancers such as malignant melanoma
- boost energy and mood, and protect against infections, such as flu.

BUT AS ALWAYS, it's the whole that determines health, not the individual parts - whether you eat a healthy diet, get enough exercise, sleep well, don't stress, don't smoke, don't drink too much alcohol. Because if these details are not respected, beta-glucans will not be a lifeline to better health.

RESISTANT STARCH

As the name suggests, 100% of resistant starch passes directly to the colon without being broken down by the body's own enzymes on the way down. Only the gut bacteria are able to break down this fibre.

There are different types of resistant starch and they are found in the hulls of cereals (whole grains), seeds, legumes, unripe bananas. Resistant starch is also found in potatoes and sweet potatoes, but when cooked (boiled, roasted, fried) starch/sugar is formed. When the potato cools, it reverts to resistant starch.

Resistant starch is a relatively unknown fibre, but it has been found to be good for building a strong intestinal lining that seals the gut against leakage, and it also helps to lower low-intensity inflammation in the body.

It is also known to counteract metabolic syndrome, over-weight and obesity.

SUMMARY: Identify which fruits, vegetables, root vegetables, mushrooms contain this fibre and which you find tasty. Then add whole grains. Eat these daily with some variety and you will build a strong microbiota that will protect you from disease. Read the chapter on Foods to avoid, so as not to break down the microbiota that is being built up.

REMEMBER that all positive effects with fibres (and other foods mentioned in the book) are only reached if you at the same time eliminate bad food and drink. You can't continue eat and drink bad products and add healthy ingre-dients and think you will reach all healthy benefits. It's like a zero sum outcome.

10

______

CEREALS

To keep it simple, I'll go through our most common grains; Wheat, Barley, Oats and Rye, including some historical and cultural varieties. The cultural varieties may have different names in other countries. Today's refined flours should be avoided if we want a healthy microbiota.

For example, wheat consists of three parts: husk, germ and flour. **All the goodness is in the husk and the germ**, while the fine flour is just empty calories.

Today's bread is bad food, but...

Bread can be both good and bad food depending on what it is made of and how it is baked. Industrial bread contains too little fibre and too much sugar. So I want to emphasise again - READ THE INGREDIENTS AND THE

NUTRITION DECLARATION on the packaging of the bread. And not just on the bread, but on ALL food you buy.

If you look at the nutrition labelling and at the carbohydrates, you will find the subgroup 'of which sugars'. If it says 20 grams, it means that the food is one fifth pure sugar.

If the product also contains additives to enhance taste and appearance such as colorings, thickeners, emulsifiers or preservatives (to extend shelf life) - don't buy!

As one nutrition expert noted, 'The longer the shelf life, the shorter the life'.

IN ADDITION to the sugar content of the product, the nutrition label will tell you the amount of dietary fibre, type of fat, protein and calories.

You'll get the best bread if you bake it yourself and use the right flours. And of course it will be even healthier and tastier if you bake with sourdough.

See under Recipes how to easily make a sourdough and how to bake bread with ancient and healthy flours.

WHEAT

There are more than 35 000 registered wheat varieties, and they are divided into two main types:

Autumn wheat, which is sown in autumn and requires a cold period to flower. Spring wheat is sown in spring and does not require a cold period to flower.

Wheat is mainly grown for its starchy seeds. The seeds have several uses, mainly as food, but also as animal feed and fuel.

Wheat grain contains gluten.

· · ·

SOME VARIETIES of wheat are Einkorn, Spelt (also known as Dinkel) and Emmer.

Wheat has been cultivated in the Middle East for at least 11 000 years.

SUBGROUPS

EINKORN OR SINGLE grain

Einkorn is the original wheat. Its name comes from the fact that it contains only one kernel in each ear. The kernels are embedded in a thick husk. Einkorn has a high nutritional content, and is resistant to many plant diseases.

The flour has a weak gluten, as in emmer and dinkel. This makes it kinder to the stomach. Unlike other more modern wheats, there is evidence that the gliadin in einkorn wheat may be less toxic to people with gluten intolerance. However, it has not yet been recommended in the gluten-free diet.

The flour is slightly yellow in color because it contains carotenoids, which are an antioxidant. Einkorn has a great aroma and flavor.

It is a nutritious wheat with a high content of protein, essential fatty acids, phosphorus, potassium, vitamin B6 and carotene.

Due to its weak gluten, a baking tin is required if you are only going to bake with einkorn flour, otherwise the dough will easily run out, resulting in a flat loaf.

EMMER WHEAT

Emmer comes from a cross between einkorn wheat and a wild grass and is also very old.

The kernels are embedded in a thick protective shell. It must be hulled before it can be milled, as with einkorn and dinkel. Emmer has a high nutritional content and its own unique flavor. Its baking properties are similar to those of einkorn.

Spelt, dinkel wheat or hulled wheat

Spelt wheat originated in south-west Asia and emerged between 6000 and 5000 BC as a result of a cross between emmer wheat and trident wheat.

Compared to common wheat flour, spelt wheat flour has a slightly higher protein content and different protein composition. Both spelt wheat and common wheat contain gluten.

Compared to common wheat, spelt has a higher protein content, a different quality of gluten, a higher proportion of healthy fatty acids and a higher energy and mineral content.

Spelt wheat contains slightly more thiamine (vitamin B1) and niacin (vitamin B3) and slightly less riboflavin (vitamin B2) compared to regular wheat.

The content of potassium and calcium is similar to that of regular wheat, while the amount of zinc, iron and copper is significantly higher in spelt wheat.

Spelt is known for its good bread aroma with a rich and slightly nutty flavor. It can be used as a substitute for wheat flour in all baked goods and dressings. Spelt flour makes a looser dough than wheat flour, so reduce the amount of yeast and let the dough rise a little longer. In addition, the bread bakes faster than bread made with wheat flour.

· · ·

BARLEY

The word barley originally referred to 'the common grain'.

Since the beginning of the Neolithic period, both naked barley, a form of six-row barley, and hulled barley have been grown in the Nordic countries. The naked grain was most common until the end of the Bronze Age, when the six-rowed hulled grain takes over. During the Late Iron Age, rye slowly began to displace barley as the main cereal. By the 16th century, barley had been displaced as the main bread grain and has since been used mainly for animal feed and malt.

Cultivated barley can be categorised into two main groups, six-row and two-row barley.

SUBGROUP:

NAKED BARLEY

It is called naked barley because the grains have loose chaff that falls off during threshing. Barley is an ancient crop that was important in the Bronze and Iron Ages and therefore belongs to the 'cultivated crops'.

During processing, many of the healthy properties of barley are normally lost, but this is not the case for naked barley, which can in principle be harvested from the field, cooked and eaten directly and is therefore much more nutritious.

Among other things, naked barley is rich in antioxidants, minerals and cholesterol-lowering beta-glucans - a soluble dietary fibre with a cholesterol-lowering effect (see chapter on Fibre).

Another good thing about barley is that the starch is broken down slowly in the stomach, so the sugar is evenly distributed in the blood, meaning there are no rapid rises in blood sugar.

A very common staple food in the Middle Ages, this 'Nordic rice' has been off the market for a long time, but has now been rediscovered and enjoyed something of a renaissance.

The fibre-rich naked grains can be cooked directly and used as a meal.

OATS

Oats have a characteristic appearance, resembling a seesaw with small stems.

One way to distinguish oats is by looking at the color of the grain; there are white, yellow and black oats.

The first oat cultivation can be traced to the Mediterranean region around 2 000 years ago.

Oats are used to make products such as oatmeal, oat mustard and various types of oat drinks and oat cream suitable for vegans and lactose intolerant people.

Oats contain a unique type of phenol - avenanthramide. This has antioxidant, anti-inflammatory and anti-atherosclerotic (prevents plaque build-up in the vascular wall) properties.

Oats contain a special fibre, beta-glucan (see chapter on Fibre), which is water-soluble and forms a gel in the gastrointestinal tract. This leads to a smoother absorption of nutrients, and oats' beta-glucan is therefore blood sugar regulating (low glycaemic index).

In several scientific studies, beta-glucans have been shown to have a cholesterol-lowering effect. Oats also contain proteins made up of various amino acids, including the amino acid tryptophan.

SUBGROUP:

NAKED OATS

This is an older unprocessed oat variety. The hulls of naked oats fall off during threshing and produce naked kernels. Naked oats contain more nutrients and energy than regular oats. It has a high quality protein, beneficial fatty acids and water-soluble fibres which stabilise blood sugar. In addition, naked oats contain high levels of vitamin E, a natural antioxidant.

Naked oats contain no gluten-forming proteins. It is also fuller and more flavorsome than regular oats. Available as flakes and whole grains.

RYE

Rye is one of the four cereals and is closely related to barley and wheat. Rye grain is used for flour, rye bread, rye beer, rye whiskey, some types of vodka and animal feed. It can also be eaten as a whole grain, either cooked or rolled, like oatmeal, or used as flour in bread baking.

Rye has been found in archaeological excavations between 1800-1500 BC. It is possible that rye came to Europe from Turkey.

Rye flour has a lower gluten content than wheat flour, and contains a higher amount of dietary fibre.

FATS - HEALTHY, UNHEALTHY AND MOST UNHEALTHY

Fat is an important source of energy for our body and the right kind of fat in the right amount is essential for our well-being.

WHY DO WE NEED FAT?

Fat provides the body with energy in a concentrated form and is stored in adipose tissue as an energy reserve. Fat insulates the body and protects our internal organs.

Fat is needed for the body to build and repair cells, and to produce hormones and hormone-like substances. Fat is also needed for the body to absorb fat-soluble vitamins A, D, E and K.

Fats also provide us with essential polyunsaturated fatty acids. These fatty acids cannot be produced by the body itself but must be obtained from food. Essential fatty acids affect a number of functions in the body, including blood pressure, blood clotting and our immune system.

. . .

HOW MUCH FAT IS ENOUGH?

Fat contains more energy than other nutrients.

1 gram (0,03 oz) of fat contains 9 calories (kcal), which is more than twice as much as a gram of carbohydrates or protein. Since fat contains a lot of energy per gram, this means that if you eat a lot of fat, you take in more energy than you expend. This can lead to overweight and obesity.

About one third of the energy you consume in a day should come from fat. For a woman, this means about 70 grams of fat per day and for a man about 90 grams.

WHICH FATS SHOULD YOU EAT?

There are different types of fat: **saturated, monounsaturated and polyunsaturated**. The difference between them is the structure of the fatty acids that make up the fat.

WITH WESTERN EATING HABITS, where much of the fat comes from meat and dairy products such as cheese, milk, sour milk, crème fraiche and butter, it's easy to get too much saturated fat and too little polyunsaturated fat. Most people would need to reduce saturated fat and increase polyunsaturated and monounsaturated fat. The fats we should eat more of are found in fish, rapeseed oil, olive oil and nuts, for example.

THERE IS ALSO a type of fat called trans fat that you should avoid. Trans fat is most often found in foods that are also high in saturated fat.

· · ·

THE FATS in food can be divided into three main groups: triglycerides, phospholipids and sterols.

TRIGLYCERIDES

Triglycerides make up the majority of the fat in our food and in our cooking fats, such as in butter, margarines and cooking oils. Most of the fat in our bodies is also made up of triglycerides, and is stored in adipose tissue.

All triglycerides are made up of a mixture of different saturated, monounsaturated and polyunsaturated fatty acids. However, the proportions are specific to different fat sources.

FOR EXAMPLE, butterfat consists of 19% monounsaturated fat, 3% polyunsaturated and 55% saturated fat.

Olive oil consists of 77% monounsaturated fat, 8% polyunsaturated and 13% saturated fat.

Rapeseed oil consists of 62% monounsaturated fat, 28% polyunsaturated and 7% saturated fatty acids.

BUTTER CONTAINS 256 mg of cholesterol while olive oil and rapeseed oil contain no cholesterol at all.

PHOSPHOLIPIDS

Phospholipids are important building blocks of cell membranes. They also help transport the fat-soluble triglycerides in the blood. A common phospholipid is lecithin, which is found in egg yolk and soya beans, for example.

· · ·

STEROLS

Sterols are a type of fat-soluble alcohol. The most common are cholesterol and various plant sterols.

CHOLESTEROL IS LARGELY FOUND ONLY in animal foods, that is, in meat and dairy products. The body also makes a lot of its own cholesterol, just over a gram a day. This is two to three times more than is normally provided by food. Cholesterol is mainly produced in the liver.

Cholesterol is needed for the body to produce the hormone cortisol, the male and female sex hormones and vitamin D. In the liver, some of the cholesterol is converted into bile acids.

PLANT STEROLS ARE similar to cholesterol but are found in foods from plants. Plant sterols reduce the amount of cholesterol absorbed in the gut. They can therefore lower the level of harmful LDL cholesterol in the blood.

Foods with added plant sterols must be specially labelled. These foods are intended for people who want to lower their blood cholesterol levels. They are less suitable for pregnant and breastfeeding women and children under five.

LIPOPROTEINS - THE TRANSPORTERS of fats

In the stomach and intestines, the fat in food is broken down into smaller particles that are absorbed in the small intestine. From there, they are transported, mainly as triglycerides and cholesterol, via the blood and lymphatic fluid to the tissues of the body. There they are converted into energy or stored in adipose tissue.

As fat is not water-soluble, fat particles are transported around the blood by blood lipids, known as lipoproteins. These are small round structures that bind to cholesterol and triglycerides.

The bad and **the good cholesterol**

There are four different types of blood lipids (lipoproteins):

Chylomicrons, Very Low Density Lipoprotein (VLDL), Low Density Lipoprotein (LDL) and High Density Lipoprotein (HDL).

Since fat is lighter than water, the more fat the lipoproteins contain, the lighter they become, hence the different names for the blood lipids.

Chylomicrons transport triglycerides from the gut to the liver and tissues.

VLDL transports triglycerides from the liver to the tissues. As the triglycerides are 'unloaded' in the body, VLDL is converted to LDL.

Most of the cholesterol in the blood is transported together with **LDL**. If there is a lot of LDL cholesterol in the blood, it can be taken up by a type of scavenger cell, called a macrophage, in the walls of the blood vessels. A build-up of these fat-filled macrophages is likely to be a major cause of atherosclerosis and clogging of blood vessels.

· · ·

BECAUSE LDL CHOLESTEROL increases the risk of atherosclerosis, which in turn increases the risk of cardiovascular disease, LDL cholesterol is often referred to as the 'bad' cholesterol.

HDL TAKES care of excess cholesterol from the cells and transports it back to the liver. In the liver, some of the cholesterol is converted into bile acids, which are emptied into the intestine via bile. The cholesterol bound to HDL is also called the 'good' cholesterol.

SATURATED, monounsaturated and polyunsaturated fatty acids

The most common fat in our bodies and in food is triglycerides. These are mostly made up of fatty acids. Fatty acids are usually divided into three groups - saturated, monounsaturated and polyunsaturated. Monounsaturated and polyunsaturated fatty acids are collectively known as unsaturated fatty acids or unsaturated fats. They are healthy fats that we should eat more of.

MONOUNSATURATED FAT

Monounsaturated fats are found in many different foods, sometimes together with saturated fats and sometimes together with polyunsaturated fats. For example, a lot of monounsaturated fat is found in:

- olive oil and olives
- rapeseed oil and edible fats made from rapeseed oil

- almonds, hazelnuts, cashew nuts and peanuts
- avocados.

How much monounsaturated **fat do we need?**

Between 10 and 20 per cent of the energy we get in a day should come from monounsaturated fat, according to the Nordic Nutrition Recommendations (NNR 2023). For a woman, this corresponds to around 30 grams and for a man just under 40 grams of monounsaturated fat per day.

The background to the recommendation is that a higher proportion of unsaturated fats in food can help reduce the risk of cardiovascular disease. Two thirds of the fat we eat should be monounsaturated and polyunsaturated.

Polyunsaturated fats

Polyunsaturated fats are essential for life. Our bodies can't make them on their own, so we need to get them from food.

What are polyunsaturated fats?

The most important polyunsaturated fats are called omega-3 and omega-6. Omega-3 and omega-6 are actually the names of two families of polyunsaturated fats.

Where are polyunsaturated fats found?

Omega-3 is found in, for example:

- oily fish such as salmon, mackerel, herring and sardines (contains EPA and DHA)
- some algae (contains EPA and DHA)
- rapeseed oil and edible fats made from rapeseed oil
- walnuts.

OMEGA-6 IS FOUND IN, for example

- corn oil
- sunflower oil, soya oil
- sesame seed and sesame seed oil
- rapeseed oil.

WHY DO we need polyunsaturated fats?

Omega-3 and omega-6 have many different functions, including helping the body to build and repair cells. They also affect the regulation of blood pressure, kidney function and our immune system.

Omega-3 reduce the blood's ability to clot, thereby reducing the risk of blood clots. For foetuses and young children, omega-3 and omega-6 are essential for normal growth and development.

Increasing the proportion of polyunsaturated fats in the diet can also help reduce the risk of cardiovascular disease.

IMPORTANCE of both omega-3 and omega-6

Omega-3 and omega-6 are often found together in the

same food. Often there is more omega-6 than omega-3 in food. Therefore, it is easier to get enough omega-6. Some foods are good sources of both omega-3 and omega-6, such as rapeseed oil and cooking fats that are high in rapeseed oil.

How much polyunsaturated **fat do we need?**

5 to 10 per cent of the energy we get from food should come from polyunsaturated fats, of which about one percentage point should come from omega-3. This corresponds to about 2.5 to 3 grams of omega-3 fats per day. That's as much omega-3 as there is in a portion of salmon or about 2 tablespoons of rapeseed oil.

One of the reasons for the Nordic Nutrition Recommendations (NNR 2023) is that the polyunsaturated fatty acids linoleic acid (omega-6) and alpha-linolenic acid (omega-3) help maintain normal blood cholesterol levels. Eating more polyunsaturated fatty acids while reducing saturated fatty acids helps reduce the risk of cardiovascular disease.

The long-chain fatty acids are important for things like foetal growth and early development.

For people who eat a mixed diet that includes fish, getting enough of the long-chain omega-3 fats DHA and EPA is rarely a problem.

For pregnant women, it is particularly important to eat oily fish once a week, as the foetus needs DHA and EPA to develop properly.

· · ·

SATURATED **fat**

Saturated fat is used as energy in the body, but it is not good for our health if too much of the fat we eat comes from saturated fat.

WHERE IS SATURATED FAT FOUND?

Saturated fat is found in animal foods and some vegetable oils, such as

- cream, ice cream and pastries
- chocolate
- fatty milk and cream
- butter and butter-based cooking fats
- cheese
- fatty meat and processed meat products such as sausages and bacon
- coconut fat and oil
- palm oil

IN GENERAL, the harder a cooking fat is in the fridge, the more saturated fat it contains.

HOW MUCH SATURATED **fat do we need?**

We don't need to eat any saturated fat at all. The saturated fatty acids needed by the body can be made from other fatty acids in food.

· · ·

ACCORDING to the Nordic Nutrition Recommendations, no more than one third of all the fat we eat, or 10% of all the energy we get, should come from saturated fat. For a woman, this corresponds to just over 20 grams (0,7 oz) and for a man around 30 grams (1,05 oz) of saturated fat per day.

The background to the recommendation is that if we eat less saturated fat it can lead to a reduced risk of cardiovascular disease if we, at the same time, eat more monounsaturated and polyunsaturated fat. Reducing saturated fat and eating more wholegrain and fibre foods is also beneficial.

TRANS fat

Consuming a lot of trans fat increases the risk of cardiovascular disease. That's why it's good that the amount of industrially produced trans fat has fallen sharply in recent years so that levels in food are now much lower.

WHAT IS TRANS FAT?

Trans fat or trans-fatty acids (TFA) is formed naturally in small amounts in ruminant animals. It can also be formed if liquid plant oils are 'partially hydrogenated'. Hardening is a technique used in the food industry to harden fats to give products the desired texture, firmness and melting point. Trans fat also increases shelf life.

If the oils are fully hardened, the unsaturated fatty acids in the oil are converted into saturated fat, if the hardening is incomplete, trans fatty acids can be formed.

HOW MUCH TRANS fat do we get?

According to the nutritional recommendations, the intake of trans fatty acids should be as low as possible.

HEALTH EFFECTS of trans fat

Trans fats increase the level of bad LDL cholesterol in the blood and reduce the level of good HDL cholesterol. This in turn increases the risk of cardiovascular disease.

Saturated fat, however, has a greater impact on the risk of cardiovascular disease because we consume 10 times more saturated fat than trans fat.

12

———

CARBOHYDRATES

Carbohydrates is the common name for starch, dietary fibre and various sugars. Carbohydrates are our main source of energy.

Sugars are fast carbohydrates that we should be careful about consuming.

Fruits, vegetables, root vegetables, legumes, whole grains are good carbohydrates that we should consume more of.

WHY DO WE NEED CARBOHYDRATES?

Most carbohydrates are broken down in the body into the sugar glucose, which is energy for the cells. Glucose is stored in the liver and muscles as glycogen, which acts as an energy reserve. The brain uses glucose as fuel and needs about 100 grams (3,5 oz) of glucose a day.

HOW CAN I choose good carbohydrates?

Science clearly shows that choosing the right type of carbohydrates is important for health. Wholegrain varieties of bread, pasta and cereals, and high-fibre foods such as vegetables, fruit and legumes have a protective effect against cancer, cardiovascular disease and type 2 diabetes. They also help maintain a healthy body weight. Therefore, the carbohydrates you eat should come primarily from these foods.

MANY PEOPLE SHOULD EAT LESS sweets, ice cream and pastries, and drink less fizzy drinks, which are high in sugar but low in nutrition.

Foods and drinks high in sugar increase the risk of getting dental caries (cavities).

If you eat foods that are high in sugar, you will find it difficult to fit in nutrient-rich foods with vitamins and minerals, without taking in more calories (energy) than you burn.

SIFTED CEREALS, which are used to make white bread and pasta, contain fewer vitamins and minerals than wholegrain flour. Eating a lot of foods based on sifted flour, sugary foods and drinks can lead to weight gain.

HOW MUCH CARBOHYDRATE IS RIGHT?

45-60% of the energy we get from food should come from carbohydrates. For someone eating 2000 kilocalories (kcal) a day, this equates to between 250 and 300 grams (8,8-10,6 oz) of carbohydrates.

· · ·

Source: Swedish National Food Agency

13
____

PROTEINS

P rotein is usually referred to as the body's building blocks. They are needed to build cells and to produce enzymes and hormones. Many people are worried about not getting enough protein. But the fact is that almost everyone gets the amount of protein they need. This is because protein is found in almost all foods, in smaller or larger amounts.

WHY DO WE NEED PROTEIN?

Protein is a component of all tissue cells in the body. In addition, hormones, enzymes and important parts of the immune system are made up of proteins. Protein is therefore essential for the functioning of the whole body.

Protein is made up of around 20 amino acids. Nine of them are essential (vital). This means that we need to get them regularly from food because the body cannot produce them on its own.

· · ·

How much protein do we need?

We get energy (calories) from fat, carbohydrates and protein and we need a good balance between these nutrients. The recommendations for adults aged 18-65 is that 10-20% of calories should come from protein. This achieves a good balance while providing you with as much protein as you need by a good margin.

As an adult, you need 0.83 g of protein per kg of body weight per day (0,03 oz per lb). If you weigh 64 kg (141 lb), you need 53 g of protein per day (1,87 oz). If you eat 2500 kilocalories (kcal) a day and follow the recommendation to get 10-20 per cent of calories from protein, you will get 63-125 g of protein per day (2,2-4,4 oz).

For those over 65, a higher intake of protein can counteract the loss of muscle mass that comes with age.

For children aged 12-23 months, the recommendation is that 10-15% of calories come from protein. This range should not be exceeded.

For children 6-11 months, the recommendation is that 7-15% of calories come from protein.

How do I get enough protein?

It is easy to get enough protein if you eat a varied diet, i.e. if you eat from all food groups. On average, 17% of calories come from protein.

Protein deficiency is rare. It only affects people who eat one-sidedly and exclude certain foods, or who get too little energy. Energy (calories) is needed for the body to use protein properly. If the body does not get enough energy, protein is used as a source of energy rather than as building blocks.

Muscles are mainly made up of protein. Many people who want to build muscle therefore eat large amounts of protein. However, eating more protein than the body needs does not automatically lead to bigger muscles. Instead, the protein can be used as an energy source and the excess energy is stored in the body's fat reserve.

Sources of protein?

Almost everyone gets the protein they need!

Protein is made up of around 20 amino acids. Nine of them are essential. We need to get these amino acids regularly from food because the body cannot produce them itself.

Foods from the animals such as meat, fish, chicken, eggs and dairy products are foods that contain all essential amino acids.

Although meat contains the essential amino acids, many people in the western world would need to eat less meat and a minimum of charcuterie (from beef, pork, game and lamb). Eating a lot of red meat and cured meats increases the risk of colorectal cancer. The current advice is not to eat more than 350 grams a week of red meat and charcuterie.

Foods from plants also almost always contain all the essential amino acids, but sometimes one or two are missing. By eating a variety of plant foods, you can get enough essential amino acids in a good mix, even without eating meat and other animal foods. What's more, essential amino acids are stored in your body when you don't need them and can be used at a later date. The body is smart and controls its needs.

Important sources of protein in plants are cereals and legumes such as peas, beans and lentils.

PROTEIN AND EXERCISE

Physical activity builds more muscle, which increases protein turnover in the muscles. Very hard exercise, especially endurance sports, also leads to an increase in muscle breakdown and the need for muscle 'repair' as a result. Therefore, it is important to get both energy (calories) and protein when exercising.

The body prefers to use fat and carbohydrates as energy sources. However, if the body does not get enough energy from fat and carbohydrates, it will use protein from food or even from muscles as an energy source. Therefore, it is important to get enough calories (fat and carbohydrates). Getting enough protein is very easy for people who are physically active because they eat a lot of food to fulfil their energy needs. And protein is found in a wide range of foods, not just those from animal sources. There is rarely a need to take supplements in the form of protein powders. However, there is a small risk of getting too little protein if you exercise while dieting.

PROTEIN FOR VEGETARIANS and vegans

It is not usually difficult for vegetarians to get enough protein, even if they exclude milk and eggs.

Beans, lentils and other legumes are good sources of plant-based protein. Other high-protein products include tofu, tempeh and other soya- or pea-based products and mycoprotein-based products.

Bread and other cereal products also contribute a lot of protein, as do nuts, seeds and vegetable drinks based on soya, for example. Those who include dairy products or eggs in their vegetarian diet naturally get a lot of readily available protein from them.

Most often, plant-based foods do not contain the essential amino acids in sufficient quantities on their own, but together they complement each other. This is called complementary action. An example is cereals and legumes. Cereals contain enough of the amino acids methionine and cysteine, which are in short supply in the legumes beans, peas and lentils. Legumes contain more of the amino acid lysine, which is not abundant in cereals. Therefore, provided you don't eat a very one-sided diet, such as rarely eating legumes, you will get enough protein even if you eat only plant-based foods.

FOR THOSE WHO TRAIN HARD, protein needs are higher. There are studies that suggest that the need among elite athletes can be as high as 1.4-1.8 grams per kilogram of body weight.

SOURCE: Swedish National Food Agency

14

LIFESTYLE DISEASES

L ifestyle diseases is a term for diseases we suffer from because of how we live. Mainly because of what we eat and don't eat, but also because we don't exercise enough and are too sedentary. And because we smoke, drink alcohol, stress and sleep too little.

DISEASES AND CONDITIONS resulting from an unhealthy lifestyle include cardiovascular diseases such as high blood pressure, high cholesterol, atrial fibrillation, heart failure, heart attack, stroke. We can also suffer from metabolic disorders such as type 2 diabetes, overweight and obesity. And gastrointestinal diseases such as IBS (irritable bowel syndrome), IBD (inflammatory bowel disease) such as Crohn's disease and ulcerative colitis. But also depression, dementia, infectious diseases due to a poor immune system. And of course cancer in all its forms.

. . .

According to the WHO (World Health Organization), a healthy lifestyle can prevent 80% of cardiovascular diseases and strokes, and 30% of all cancers. Healthy lifestyles can also prevent or delay the development of type 2 diabetes.

Our genes account for about 10% of the risk to develop diseases that our parents pass on to us. Whether we get ill or not is is to a very large extent determined by our lifestyle.

It is also not normal to be frail and get diseases at the age of 70. In the vast majority of cases, it is a consequence of how we have lived our lives.

Here is a brief description of lifestyle diseases and what each condition means:

High blood pressure (hypertension)
The journey of blood in the body both begins and ends in the heart. It is pumped out into the body from the left ventricle of the heart (= systolic blood pressure) and received in the right atrium of the heart (= diastolic blood pressure). This is called the systemic circulation. There is also a pulmonary circulation, which means that when the blood returns to the right atrium of the heart, it is pumped to the right ventricle and on to the lungs to leave carbon dioxide and other products the body wants to get rid of and pick up new oxygen, before being pumped back to the heart and further out into the body.

High blood pressure is considered to be 140/90 or higher, where the high value is the systolic pressure (blood pumping out into the body) and the low is the diastolic pressure (blood coming back to the heart). High blood pressure can be caused by many factors, but this section only discusses lifestyle as a cause.

Blood vessels become stiff and a higher resistance occurs. The stiffness of the vessels can be caused by the food we eat and the build-up of blood fats (cholesterol) in the vessel wall, but also by smoking, alcohol and lack of exercise.

High blood pressure increases the risk of secondary diseases such as stroke, heart attack, heart failure, kidney disease, dementia and poor circulation in the legs.

BLOOD LIPIDS

There are two main types of fats in the blood - cholesterol and triglycerides.

Triglycerides are used by the body as a source of energy, while cholesterol is needed to build cells and produce different types of hormones. We get some cholesterol from our diet, but most of it is made in the body. If we get too much of these fats in our blood, they can be stored in the liver or lodge in the walls of blood vessels, which increases the risk of cardiovascular disease.

HDL CHOLESTEROL: There are different types of cholesterol carrier proteins in the blood. High density lipoprotein (HDL) cholesterol is also known as 'good cholesterol' as it removes excess cholesterol.

LDL CHOLESTEROL: Low density lipoprotein (LDL) cholesterol is also known as 'bad cholesterol'. High levels of

LDL cholesterol are associated with an increased risk of developing various types of cardiovascular diseases.

APOLIPOPROTEIN B (APO B): is the carrier protein of LDL cholesterol, as well as of other harmful fat particles such as VLDL (VeryLowDensityLipoprotein) and IDL (semi-high density, composed mainly of triglycerides and cholesteryl esters) which are associated with an increased risk of cardiovascular disease. High levels of Apo B are associated with an increased risk of developing various types of cardiovascular disease such as heart attack and stroke.

APOLIPOPROTEIN A1 (APO A1): is the carrier protein of HDL cholesterol, also known as 'good cholesterol'. Deficiency of Apolipoprotein A1 or HDL cholesterol can lead to an increased risk of cardiovascular disease.

TRIGLYCERIDES: we get these mainly from the food we eat. If we get too much of this fat in our blood, it can be stored in the liver or in the walls of blood vessels, which can increase the risk of cardiovascular disease.

LIPOPROTEIN(A), Lp(a): is a variant of LDL cholesterol that was described as early as the 1980s as being associated with an increased risk of cardiovascular disease. The Lp(a) particle consists of an LDL particle linked to a specific peptide, apolipoprotein(a), apo(a). An increased risk of cardiovascular disease is present at elevated levels. The concentration in the blood is strongly linked to heredity and elevated Lp(a) should be characterised as a genetic disorder.

Current European guidelines recommend that Lp(a) should be included in cardiovascular risk assessment, at least once for each person.

Atrial fibrillation (AF)

In atrial fibrillation, the heart rhythm is not controlled by the normal impulse generator in the heart (the sinus node), but is instead controlled by electrical chaos in the atrium of the heart, which causes the heart to pump irregularly. As the atria do not contribute to the work of the heart in atrial fibrillation, the function of the heart is more or less impaired, and this can be exacerbated if the heart rate is too high for a long time. Many people experience it as if they have reduced fitness.

The cause of atrial fibrillation is often linked to other diseases that affect the heart, especially high blood pressure, which is present in the majority of patients with atrial fibrillation.

The risk of atrial fibrillation is also strongly linked to older age. This is probably because an unhealthy lifestyle over many years eventually leads to AF.

Obesity, inactivity and high alcohol consumption are factors that increase the risk of AF. Atrial fibrillation can also affect people who are otherwise healthy.

Atrial fibrillation almost never poses an acute threat to circulation, but it does increase the risk of heart failure, stroke and is also associated with dementia.

The symptoms of atrial fibrillation vary widely and can include palpitations, a bubbling sensation in the chest, shortness of breath, dizziness, fatigue, chest pain and reduced fitness.

Heart failure

In heart failure, the heart's ability to work is reduced and the heart is no longer able to pump enough blood around the body to oxygenate and nourish the body's cells. The heart grows so it can manage to pump blood into the body. The chambers enlarge and the pumping ability deteriorates.

You may have right-sided heart failure, in which case the blood may pool in the legs, which become swollen, or left-sided heart failure, in which case the blood pools in the lungs instead. When the heart is no longer able to pump the blood out of the body at the rate it should, there is a 'queue' of blood and this queue ends up in the lungs in left-sided failure, which can lead to pulmonary edema. In simple terms, in pulmonary edema you get fluid in the lungs (the blood is largely made up of fluid) and it is like drowning, but the fluid comes from inside. This only happens in advanced heart failure.

Symptoms of heart failure include tiredness, shortness of breath at rest or on exertion and leg swelling. In the case of pulmonary edema, you may find it difficult to breathe.

Causes of heart failure include prolonged high blood pressure, atrial fibrillation or damage to the heart from one or more heart attacks.

Myocardial infarction

Acute myocardial infarction is usually caused by the build-up of cholesterol (plaque) in the walls of the coronary arteries (which oxygenate the heart). The vessel becomes increasingly narrow until the blood can no longer pass through and it stops.

Typical symptoms include chest discomfort/pressure/pain, sometimes radiating to one or both arms, the neck, the jaw and/or between the shoulder blades. Nausea, dizziness, shortness of breath (breathlessness) and cold sweats may also occur. Symptoms such as back pain can also occur before you have a heart attack so you need to be alert to any new symptoms and take them seriously. A slow clogging of the vessels can cause angina and cause symptoms (back or chest pain) when you exert yourself. Always call 112 without delay if you experience these symptoms.

Stroke (clot/haemorrhage)

In a stroke, blood flow to a part of the brain is interrupted or severely reduced. This can lead to the damage or death of brain cells, which can cause loss of neurological functions. In about 10% of cases, the cause is haemorrhage and in about 90%, a blood clot. In principle, a stroke is always an acute illness.

Symptoms of stroke can vary depending on the part of the brain affected and the severity of the damage. Common symptoms include sudden paralysis, usually in one half of the body, numbness in the face, arms or legs, confusion, difficulty speaking or understanding speech, vision problems and headaches.

Common risk factors are high blood pressure, atrial fibrillation, smoking, excessive alcohol consumption. Always call 112 if you experience these symptoms.

· · ·

IBS

Irritable Bowel Syndrome (IBS), is a malfunction between the gut and the brain. A growing body of evidence suggests that the cause is a dysbiosis in the gut microbiota. The bacteria of the microbiota communicate with other organs through so-called 'axes' and in this case with the brain. You may also be intolerant to certain foods.

Typical symptoms of IBS include abdominal pain (which often increases after eating but eases after emptying the bowel), irregular bowel movements, changes in the consistency of stools, gas and a 'bloated' stomach. Note that similar symptoms can also be a sign of cancer so it must be ruled out.

Treatment should start by changing your diet for 4-8 weeks and trying a FODMAP diet. FODMAP is an abbreviation for Fermentable, Oligo-, Di-, Mono-saccharides and Polyols, i.e. carbohydrates that are not fermented.

Examples of low FODMAP foods that do not irritate the stomach are:

Vegetables: Carrots, green beans, potatoes, tomato and cucumber.

Fruit: Banana, blueberries, orange and melon.

Cereals: Rice, oats, quinoa and corn.

Dairy products: Lactose-free products, hard cheeses (e.g. cheddar).

Protein: Chicken, fish, eggs and tofu.

INFLAMMATORY BOWEL DISEASE (IBD)

IBD is an umbrella term for inflammatory bowel diseases, with Crohn's disease and ulcerative colitis being the most common. The cause of IBD is unclear but is thought to be multifactorial with genetic, environmental and microbiological factors. It has also been found that a dysbiosis in the microbiota can cause the diseases and that a high-fibre diet can improve symptoms.

CROHN'S DISEASE can affect the entire gastrointestinal tract from the oral cavity to the rectum, but most commonly affects the lower part of the small intestine, colon and rectum. Symptoms include diarrhoea, sometimes with blood and mucus, abdominal pain, weight loss, malnutrition.

ULCERATIVE COLITIS AFFECTS the colon and rectum. Symptoms include diarrhoea with blood and mucus, abdominal pain when emptying the bowel, frequent diarrhoea, systemic effects such as fever, rapid pulse and low blood pressure.

DEPRESSION

Depression is a very common disorder characterised by low mood, anxiety, psychomotor retardation, difficulty sleeping and loss of appetite. Depression is common and is one of the major diseases of our time. Almost one third of the population will experience depression at some point in their lives. Depression can be categorised into different types (for more information, search online).

Studies have shown a link between depression and a dysbiosis in the gut microbiota.

DEMENTIA / Alzheimer's

Dementia is caused by damage to the brain and can manifest itself in different ways depending on which parts are affected. Memory and the ability to plan and carry out everyday tasks are usually impaired. Language, time perception and orientation are other so-called cognitive functions that are negatively affected.

Anxiety, depression and behavioral changes can also be part of the disease picture. Taken together, these symptoms make it difficult to cope with life without support from others. Dementia is much more common in old age, but it does not affect everyone and is not a natural part of aging.

By far the most common dementia is Alzheimer's disease, which accounts for 60-70% of all cases.

Sometimes depression in older people can be confused with dementia.

CANCER

There are around 200 different types of cancers. Cancer means that the balance in a cell is disturbed. A previously healthy cell starts to misbehave. It doesn't know when to stop dividing. The new cells - the cancer cells - do not do their job properly. They continue to divide unchecked. More and more cancer cells are formed. And after a while, they become a small clump of cells - a tumor has formed. The tumor continues to grow. Eventually it is so big that you can see or feel it.

Symptoms of cancer may include a lump in the breast or elsewhere on the body, sores that don't heal, abnormal bleeding, coughing or hoarseness that won't go away, difficulty swallowing, change in bowel habits or difficulty peeing, new or a changed mole.

Common cancers are Prostate cancer, Breast cancer,

Skin cancer (malignant melanoma is the most aggressive), Colorectal cancer (fourth most common type, the number of cases is increasing and alarmingly also among younger people), Lung cancer (increasingly common among women), Bladder cancer (more common among men).

About 40% of all cancers and almost half of all deaths are linked to preventable lifestyle factors, according to the latest scientific reports. And a not so wild guess is that the correlation between our lifestyle and other cancer types will be found in the near future.

TYPE 2 DIABETES

About 5% of a European population has diabetes, of which about 90% is type 2 diabetes. As we become more obese, these numbers will probably increase in the coming years.

In type 2 diabetes, the ability to produce insulin is not completely gone but the amount of insulin is not enough for the body's needs. Many people with type 2 diabetes are overweight, and obesity is one of the reasons why body cells lose their sensitivity to insulin.

Early in the course of the disease, symptoms are few, with no or mild distress. Later in the disease, symptoms are more pronounced and can lead to complications of varying severity. Symptoms may include increased thirst, frequent urination, both physical and mental fatigue, repeated fungal infections e.g. genital, foot ulcers, numbness in hands and feet, visual impairment.

OVERWEIGHT / obesity

Overweight and obesity is a risk factor for a number of

diseases and is one of the main causes of bad health, lost healthy years and premature death.

Being overweight is a condition that can increase the risk of developing obesity. Obesity is a chronic disease that often requires long-term treatment and follow-up.

Being overweight or obese increases the risk of type 2 diabetes, cancer, cardiovascular disease, but also social stigmatization and its consequences.

For overweight and obese children and adolescents, there is a high risk that overweight and obesity will persist into adulthood, and that it will affect physical and mental health. For pregnant women, in addition to the personal health risks, overweight and obesity also increase the risk of pregnancy and labour complications and have a negative impact on the baby.

OVERWEIGHT AND OBESITY are increasing in all age groups.

THE ABSOLUTE BEST method for weight loss is to never gain weight. Evolution has designed us to economise on calories. Historically, there has been a shortage of food, so the body has the ability to switch off the burning of calories. For this reason, it is difficult to lose weight. And I would say that you will never lose weight just by exercising. For that to happen, you need to walk at least 5 hours a day at a fast pace and in hilly terrain. I dare to say this because I have walked several pilgrimage routes in Spain, the longest of which was 800 km and partly in hilly terrain. During the 29 days of walking, I lost about 3-4 kilos (6,5-9 lb) and probably mostly as liquid. It was quick to regain the original weight.

. . .

You NEED to change your diet to have a successful weight loss and a sustainable weight.

IT IS ALSO QUITE common to reward yourself after exercise with something that may not be very healthy. The few calories you just burned are then immediately returned.

STUDIES HAVE ALSO CONCLUDED that there is no such thing as healthy obesity.

THE OBESITY EPIDEMIC - BACKGROUND

Like so many other things, the obesity epidemic started in the USA. Partly through political decisions and partly through the stockbrokers on Wall Street and their ever-increasing demands for corporate returns. Both on food producers and on food chains.

WE CAN PROBABLY PLACE a large part of the blame and responsibility on the same actors for the ongoing obesity epidemic we have in Europe and other continents. As we are following the trends from the US.

THE BACKGROUND

The unprecedented increase in the power, scale and sophistication of food marketing, which started around 1980, is closely aligned with the explosion of the obesity epidemic.

· · ·

In the 1970s, the US government went from subsidize only a few of the bad foods, to paying companies to produce many more of them. The US Congress passed laws that, contrary to the laws in place to support a long-term agricultural policy, aimed at protecting prices by limiting production, instead started paying out money in proportion to production. The more that was produced, the higher the payout. Extra calories began to flow into the food supply.

In 1981, General Electric CEO Jack Welch gave a speech in which he launched General Electric's 'shareholder value movement', which directed companies' primary goal towards maximizing short-term returns for investors. In this way, Wall Street put pressure on food companies to present increased profits and growth every quarter to boost their share price.

There was already an abundance of calories on the market and now they had to sell even more.

This put companies in a difficult position. Food producers could no longer choose to produce the healthy products even if they wanted to. They are dependent on investors. If they stopped marketing to children, or tried to sell healthier food, or did anything else that could jeopardize their short-term profits, Wall Street would demand a change in corporate management. Healthy products are bad for business. It's not a conspiracy, it's not even anyone's fault. It's just the way the market works.

Given the constant demands for corporate growth and quick returns in an already oversaturated market, the food industry needed to get people to eat more. Like the tobacco industry before them, the food industry turned to the advertising agencies. The food industry spends about $10 billion a year on advertising and another $20 billion on other forms of marketing, such as trade shows, consumer campaigns, lobbying and so-called 'slotting fees' at grocery stores.

FOOD AND BEVERAGE companies purchase shelf space (slotting fees) in supermarkets to clearly display their most profitable products. The method forces suppliers to outbid each other for the shelf space. The practice is also known as "cliffing," because companies "force suppliers to bid against each other for shelf space with the loser pushed 'over the cliff.'" Since these fees can cost up to $20,000 per item, per store and per city, you can imagine the types of foods that producers pay to sell. And it's not cauliflower.

To GET an idea of the types of products that get the prime spots, just go to the checkout aisle. You will find sweets and drinks. Just by increasing sales by 1 per cent, a store can earn an extra $15,000 a year. Let's remember that the primary goal of food businesses (producers and suppliers) is to make money. Not to support their customers health.

For example, tens of millions of dollars are spent annually to promote a single candy product. McDonald's alone can spend billions of dollars a year. Today, the food industry is the industry that spends the most money on advertising.

REAGAN'S DEREGULATION policy removed the ban on TV advertising of food products to children. Today, the average child can see more than 10,000 food advertisements a year, in addition to online, print, cinema, video games, or on their mobile phones. Almost all food and drink adverts for children globally are products that negatively affect their health.

In addition to the early exposure to advertising, food marketing has become very sophisticated. With the help of psychologists, companies began to understand what factors unconsciously influence sales. For example, they found out how to influence children and get them to manipulate their parents.

Packaging was designed to best capture a child's attention, and then these products are placed at eye level in the store. The mirror bubbles on the ceiling of supermarkets are not just for detecting shoplifters. Cameras and GPS-like devices on shopping trolleys are used to create strategies on how best to guide customers towards the most profitable products on the market. Behavioral psychology is widely used to increase impulse purchases, and eye movement tracking technology is used.

OVERWEIGHT AND OBESITY

You probably have a pretty good idea of how much money you have in your bank account by looking at the balance from time to time.

If you feel sick, you might measure your body temperature.

When you drive your car, you probably look at the speed sometimes. And follows the route in the navigator.

THESE THREE EXAMPLES are about feedback. Feedback is essential if you want to know where you are and if you are following your route. And you need to get feedback continuously.

Therefore, you should also check your weight from time to time. You can also measure your abdominal circumference.

And be aware of the following - when you're fully grown, **it's never the clothes that are too small.** It is you who has grown. The most effective way to deal with your weight gain is to address it immediately and not start buying bigger clothes. Because once you start, you will continue.

THE MOST COMMON cause of overweight and obesity is eating more calories (energy) than you burn. Then there are big differences between individuals in how much excess weight you put on. If two people eat exactly the same amount and one has genes that keep them slim, that person will not gain as much weight as a person without slim genes. You can inherit obesity genes from your parents, but the likelihood of you becoming obese if your parents feed your child a nutritious, healthy, low-calorie diet is obviously small. Having overweight parents does not automatically mean that you will become overweight yourself. You control your weight through what you eat and how much you exercise.

Being overweight often leads to risk factors such as high cholesterol, high blood pressure and high blood sugar. But even a slim person who eats an unhealthy diet can suffer from it.

ACCORDING TO THE WHO, in 2022, 43% of adults aged 18 years and over were overweight and 16% were living with obesity. In the USA more than two-thirds of adults are overweight or have obesity. Similar trends can also be seen in younger age groups.

By 2050, the total number of children, adolescents and adults with overweight and obesity will reach over 250 million (The Lancet).

The proportion of children who are overweight is also increasing, which is worrying because children have also been found to have high blood pressure, high cholesterol and high blood sugar. It has also been shown that children may have difficulty normalizing these risk factors even if they become normal weight. Therefore, it is important to prevent children from becoming overweight.

As WEIGHT GAIN usually occurs gradually and over time, it can be difficult to detect when it happens. However, it is important to address it immediately when it happens. We humans have a tendency to compare ourselves to people who are a little worse off than we are - like someone who smokes more than I do, someone drinks more than I do, someone is more overweight than I am. Therefore I allow myself to continue to eat and drink unhealthily for a while longer. 'I SHALL lose weight, but I do it 'tomorrow'.

A common statement from overweight people is 'I've really tried EVERYTHING to lose weight'. This is definitely not true. You might have tried a lot, but certainly not everything and definitely not for long enough. It has taken years to gain weight. Losing weight will take a long time too - the more kilos or pounds you put on, the longer it takes to get rid of them. Patience and perseverance are essential to lose weight and to achieve sustainable weight loss.

A FEW IMPORTANT things to emphasize:
1. There is no such thing as healthy overweight

Studies have shown that you get fitter by exercising, which is good, but you don't get rid of the risk factors associated with obesity such as high blood pressure (exercise can lower it slightly), cholesterol, inflammation markers (C-reactive protein, CRP), insulin resistance (exercise affects insulin resistance), HbA1c (Haemoglobin A1c, correlates well with the risk of developing diabetes complications). Note that not all overweight people have all risk markers.

One study found that compared to people with a healthy weight, those with obesity (who did not smoke, did not drink too much alcohol, engaged in physical activity and ate a good diet) were at higher risk of several diseases regardless of whether they achieved high lifestyle scores. However, healthy obese people had a lower risk of lifestyle diseases compared to obese adults who were not healthy.

2. You won't lose weight just by walking or jogging

You need to reduce your energy intake. If you exercise, you are also likely to get hungrier or reward yourself for being good. It is human nature to reward yourself when you have performed a physical activity and you should do so. But not with high-calorie products.

I have walked 3 pilgrimage routes in Spain, most recently in 2022 when I walked the Camino Primitivo for 13 days.

It is 325 km (202 miles) and very hilly with a total of 7000 metres (7650 yd) of altitude. I did not lose many kilos or pounds. During a one-day stage you burn 1600-1700 calories (according to the training app). Probably more because you are hiking with excess weight in your backpack weighing 4-5 kg (9-11 pounds) and a few litres of water. You need to replenish your energy continuously to be able to hike 30 km (19 mi) per day in hilly terrain. At the finish line, I had only lost 3-4 kg (7-9 lb). The daily temperature was around 35 degrees Celsius (95 °F) so most of the lost

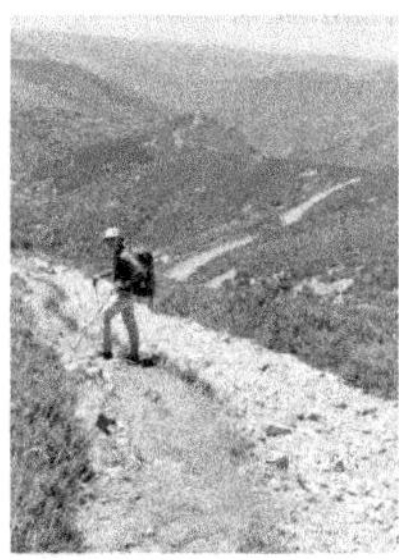

Hospitales is one of the most beautiful stages during the Camino Primitivo (2022).

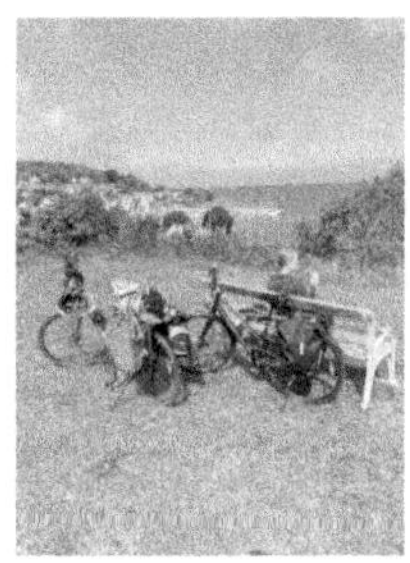

Lunch break in Arild in southwest of Sweden (2023)

kilos was probably body fluid, because I quickly returned to my original weight.

I have also holidayed by bike.

When you cycle for 5-6 hours, you burn more calories than when you walk for the same hours. In addition, cycling does not put as much strain on the body (feet, knees, back). That's why I recommend cycling over walking as exercise. But the best exercise is of course the one that gets done!

3. The body is not designed to lose weight

Throughout our evolution, we have been mostly exposed to lack of food, so when starvation occurs, the body slows down the metabolism. If you are overweight and start exercising, you will lose a few kilos fairly immediately. But after a short while, you stop losing weight. Your body works against you by switching off the metabolism. Therefore, you have to try to trick your body by alternating between jogging and walking, or walking alternately slow and fast, or walking on hilly terrain, so that your body does not recognise the exercise pattern. Another way might be to exercise at different times of the day.

4. The microbiota can help you lose weight

The lower part of your intestine produces hormones that tell your gut to slow down bowel movements and it also helps to influence metabolism and appetite. One of these hormones is GLP-1. The new weight loss medicines use a synthetic variant, semaglutide or tirzepatide, to trigger the same effect.

So you can stimulate your gut to produce these hormones naturally, by fueling your gut bacteria with the food you eat.

To conclude - you MUST change your diet to lose weight.

Obesity and cancer

The link between weight and cancer may not be linear, but large-scale epidemiological studies have shown a consistent and convincing association between obesity and the risk of developing cancer.

Studies also show that obesity reduces life expectancy by up to 8 years and is linked to at least 236 medical problems, including 13 types of cancer.

The following cancers are linked to obesity:

- Oesophageal cancer
- Colorectal cancer
- Gallbladder cancer
- Stomach cancer
- Liver cancer
- Pancreatic cancer
- Breast cancer (especially menopausal women)
- Uterine cancer
- Kidney cancer
- Ovarian cancer
- Thyroid cancer
- Meningioma (arising from the membranes of the brain or spinal cord)
- Multiple myeloma

As you can see, several cancers are directly related to the transport of food through the intestines. Of course, the cancer may also be related to the food you eat.

Chronic inflammation is a characteristic of obesity and is a known cause of cancer. In addition, insulin resistance, hyperglycemia (high blood sugar) and dyslipidaemia (high blood lipids) resulting from obesity can influence tumor growth and cancer development.

Better gut health can lead to weight loss

Injectable drugs for weight loss have received a lot of attention recently. As mentioned earlier, an alternative route to medication for weight loss may be to improve the gut microbiota (all the billions of micro-organisms that live in the gut - read more in the chapter on the microbiota).

Humans need to have a diversity of microorganisms in our gut, especially in the large intestine (colon). Gut bacteria feed on fibre from the food we eat and convert fibre into substances that the body needs. These substances communicate with other organs by sending signals.

A dysbiosis in the microbiota can affect these signals, leading to health problems such as inflammatory bowel disease, autoimmune diseases, diabetes, cardiovascular diseases, asthma.

Ultra-processed foods, which contain many additives, such as thickeners, emulsifiers, colorings and preservatives, can lead to a serious dysbiosis in the microbiota.

People with obesity have less diverse microbiota. Animal studies have shown that when normal-weight mice were fed gut bacteria from obese mice, they gained weight.

In another study, when subjects were given a diet designed more to provide energy to the gut bacteria than to the body, the subjects lost some weight.

CHILDREN INHERIT THEIR PARENTS' obesity

Results from the Tromsø Study (an ongoing Norwegian population-based health study), found that the odds of children being obese in middle age are six times higher if both parents were obese in middle age, compared to if both parents were normal weight (BMI 18.5-24.9). If only one parent was obese, the child was about 3.5 times more likely to be obese in middle age.

WEIGHT FLUCTUATIONS INCREASE the risk of cardiovascular disease

One study found that fluctuate in weight is associated

with an increased risk of cardiovascular events (27% increased risk), cardiovascular death (29% increased risk), heart attack (32% increased risk), stroke (21% increased risk).

Pregnancy

According to the Public Health Agency of Sweden, the prevalence of overweight (BMI over 25) or obesity (BMI over 30) in pregnant women at the time of enrolment in antenatal care increased from 25% in 1992 to 46% in 2022.

The risk of preterm birth is three times higher for women with obesity.

A report from the National Board of Health and Welfare shows that pregnant women with a high BMI ($\geq$ 25) were more likely to have pre-eclampsia, high blood pressure and gestational diabetes than those of normal weight.

Caesarean sections were more common in overweight and obese pregnant women, and a greater proportion of these sections were emergency.

Repeated miscarriages were almost twice as common in pregnant women with a BMI $\geq$ 30 compared to those of normal weight. The incidence was highest in women in the highest obesity class (BMI $\geq$ 40).

Newborns whose mothers were overweight or obese during pregnancy were more likely to have breathing problems, low blood sugar and a low Apgar score < 7 at 5 minutes (Apgar is a model used to measure the health of newborns at 1, 5 and 10 minutes after birth, the higher the score the better the health and higher the chances of survival) compared to newborns with normal weight mothers.

High birth weights $\geq$ 4500 g were also more common,

increasing the risk of complications. Stillbirth, which is rare in itself, was more common in babies born to obese women (BMI ≥ 30) compared to normal weight women.

Long-term follow-up showed that babies born to women with a high BMI (BMI ≥ 30) were more likely to develop asthma, suffer from infections and have bowel dysfunction compared to babies born to normal weight mothers. The higher the BMI of the mother, the higher the percentage of children with these diagnoses. There were also more children diagnosed with obesity, ADHD and autism spectrum disorders.

17

____

FOOD ADDITIVES

Emulsifiers, stabilisers, thickeners and gelling agents (solidifiers) are a group of food additives used to affect the texture of a product, among other things.

In addition to these, there are colorings and sweeteners that allow the producer to change a product to look more appealing but also to have a higher sweetness. Add fat (often bad fat) and together with the above additives we have created an ultra-processed product that is made to be hard to resist.

THERE IS A GROWING body of research on food additives and how they affect our health. Recently, there have been reports of emulsifiers destroying the microbiota. And that's something you should avoid if you want to keep your health.

A large study published in 2024 showed a link between the consumption of certain emulsifiers and an increased risk of certain cancers, particularly breast and prostate cancer.

Emulsifiers have also been linked to an increased risk of cardiovascular disease.

Read the list of ingredients on the food you buy and avoid products with emulsifiers and other additives. The more substances, the worse.

Emulsifiers

Emulsifiers are so-called surfactants. This means that they have the ability to reduce the surface tension between two substances that cannot actually mix.

Emulsifiers are used to allow one substance to diffuse into the other, making the mixture stable. If these substances are liquids, such as oil and water, the result is called an emulsion. Milk is an example of an emulsion where fat is distributed in water.

Emulsifiers can also be used to facilitate the production of certain foods and to preserve properties during transport and storage. Emulsifiers affect viscosity (inertia), appearance, structure, texture (chewing resistance).

Lecithin is an example of a common emulsifier.

Emulsifiers occur naturally in many foods and are extracted from their natural sources. Others are semi-synthetic or fully synthetic.

Stabilising agents

It is difficult to specify exactly which substances belong to the group of stabilisers. This is partly because thickeners, emulsifiers and other additives also often have a stabilising function in different ways.

For example, stabilisers can be used to prevent the strawberries from floating to the surface of the strawberry jam.

· · ·

THICKENING AND GELLING agents

Thickening and gelling agents typically dissolve or disperse in water to form a viscous solution or gel. This is what makes them useful in the food industry.

These substances are used to make products that are too thin, such as ketchup, more viscous. Many are derived from natural sources, such as potato and rice flours, and have long been used for various purposes. More recently, chemically modified forms of natural substances, such as certain species of algae, have also been used.

MODIFIED starches

Starch is a food raw material, but if it is modified by a chemical process, it is considered an additive. Depending on the chemical process used, different properties are obtained.

The declaration of modified starches must be supplemented by an indication of the specific plant species from which it has been produced and whether the modified starch may contain gluten.

SOURCE. Swedish National Food Agency

NUTRITION LABELLING - INGREDIENT LIST

By far the best tool we have to check whether what we eat and drink is good or bad for us is the Ingredient list and Nutrition labelling on all products. From these you can determine the content, calories and nutrients such as fat (total and saturated fat), protein, carbohydrates (total and how much sugar), salt and fibre (see below) and additional content if the producer chooses to display it, such as vitamins and minerals.

Nutrition labelling (per 100 g / 3,5 oz or 100 ml / 0,4 cups) is mandatory on pre-packaged foods (with some exceptions).

The purpose of nutrition labelling is to provide consumers with a standardized way of obtaining information on the energy and nutrient content of different foods.

Nutrition labelling describes how much energy and which nutrients, and how much of them, a food contains.

· · ·

MANDATORY INFORMATION in the nutrition labelling is information on the energy value and amount of

- fat
  - of which saturated fat
- carbohydrate
  - of which sugars
- protein
- salt

OTHER NUTRIENTS, which may be listed voluntarily in the nutrition declaration are

- monounsaturated fat
- polyunsaturated fat
- polyols
- starch
- fibre
- vitamins and minerals

HERE ARE some examples of the nutritional content of foods.

WHITE RICE - very low in fibre and high in (fast) carbohydrates - bad for the microbiota and raises blood sugar.

· · ·

Nutrition information per 100 g (3,5 oz)
Energy 1487 kJ, 350 kcal
Fat 0.7 g (0,02 oz)
Of which saturated fat 0.3 g (0,01 oz)
Carbohydrate 79 g (2,8 oz)
Of which sugars 0.2 g (0,007 oz)
Protein 7.1 g (0,25 oz)
Salt 0 g
Fibre 0.5 g (0,018 oz)

BLACK RICE - CONTAINS SIGNIFICANTLY MORE fibre and minerals than white rice due to the fact that it is a whole grain rice with the innermost husk of the grain still attached.

Nutritional value per 100 g (3,5 oz)
Energy content
- 1400 kJ/330 kcal
Fat 3.4 g (0,12 oz)
of which saturated fat 0.9 g (0,03 oz)
Carbohydrate 64 g (2,26 oz)
of which sugars 1.2 g (0,04 oz)
Fibre 8.5 g (0,3 oz)
Protein 9.9 g (0,35 oz)
Salt <0.02 g** (0,0007 oz)
Phosphorus 282 mg 40% (0,01 oz)
Magnesium 115 mg 31%* (0,004 oz)
Selenium 14 µg 25%
Zinc 2.1 mg 21%* (0,0007 oz)
* of DRI (daily reference intake)
** The salt content is exclusively due to naturally occur-

ring sodium.

VEGO MINCE - frozen soya mince made from soya protein. Compare the content with the cold pressed mince below.

NUTRITIONAL INFORMATION per 100 g (3,5 oz)
Energy 780 kJ, 186 kcal
Fat 9.8 g (0,35 oz)
Of which saturated fat 0.8 g (0,028 oz)
Carbohydrate 4.6 g (0,16 oz)
Of which sugars 1.1 g (0,039 oz)
Protein 17 g (0,6 oz)
Salt 0.73 g (0,026 oz)
Fibre 5.2 g (0,18 oz)

VEGGIE MINCE - from cold-pressed soya beans. Contains much more protein, more fibre and less salt than frozen soybean meal. Is not processed at all, but contains only soybeans, unlike the frozen alternatives.

NUTRITIONAL INFORMATION per 100 g (3,5 oz)
Energy 1688 kJ, 400 kcal
Fat 8.5 g (0,3 oz)
Of which saturated fat 1.5 g (0,05 oz)
Carbohydrate 32 g (1,13 oz)
Of which sugars 9 g (0,32 oz)
Protein 47 g (1,66 oz)
Salt 0 g

Fibre 16 g (0,56 oz)

BUTTER - is high in saturated fat, which we should avoid and don't need to eat at all according to the Swedish National Food Agency (see chapter on Fats)

NUTRITIONAL INFORMATION per 100 g (3,5 oz)
Energy 3038 kJ, 739 kcal
Fat 82 g (2,9 oz)
Of which saturated fat 52 g (1,8 oz)
Of which monounsaturated fat 20 g (0,7 oz)
Of which polyunsaturated fat 1.9 g (0,07 oz)
Carbohydrate 0.7 g (0,02 oz)
Of which sugars 0.7 g (0,02 oz)
Protein 0.6 g (0,02 oz)
Salt 0.2 g (0,007 oz)
Fibre 16 g (0,56 oz)
Cholesterol 0.25 g (0,009 oz)

EXTRA VIRGIN olive oil - is probably the best fat for us, and is the most studied fat included in the Mediterranean diet. It should be extra virgin because it contains all the beneficial substances such as polyphenols (a type of antioxidant that protects against cancer and against rancidity), and is also a good source of essential fatty acids such as omega 3 and omega 6. Personally, I use olive oil on my breakfast sandwiches instead of butter or margarine.

NUTRITIONAL INFORMATION per 100 g (3,5 oz)

Energy 3700 kJ, 900 kcal
Fat 100 g (3,5 oz)
Of which saturated fat 14 g (0,5 oz)
Of which monounsaturated fat 73 g (2,5 oz)
Of which polyunsaturated fat 12 g (0,4 oz)
Cholesterol 0 g

INGREDIENTS

Food and drink products must also list their ingredients. In the list of ingredients, ingredients must be listed in descending order of quantity (there are some exceptions). Each ingredient must be properly labelled with its specific name. Additives, flavorings and enzymes are also ingredients that must be listed.

As a general rule, all ingredients used to make a food must be listed in the list of ingredients.

HERE ARE some examples of ingredients used in foods and snacks.

NOTE - these are products found in Swedish grocery stores. They are examples and you can find similar products in your store if you look at the ingredient list.

MALLEABLE VEGGIE MINCE - WATER, SOY protein (23%), rapeseed oil, onion, salt, spices, apple extract, natural flavor, stabilizer (methyl cellulose).

COLD PRESSED veggie mince (same as mentioned above

under nutritional content) - SOY mince from cold pressed SOY beans (no additives beyond that).

MILK CHOCOLATE (MARABOU) - SUGAR, cocoa butter, cocoa mass, whey powder (MILK), SKIMMED MILK POWDER, BUTTER FAT, whey product (MILK), emulsifier (SOY lecithin), flavoring. Minimum 30% cocoa.

An ultra-processed product that contains additives that make you addicted to it but also emulsifier that is harmful to the microbiota.

70% dark chocolate (Marabou) - Cocoa mass, sugar, cocoa butter, fat-reduced cocoa, butterfat, emulsifier (soya lecithin), flavoring, skimmed milk powder. Minimum 70% cocoa.

This Marabou product contains additives, including an emulsifier that is harmful to the microbiota.

70% dark chocolate (Lindt) - cocoa mass, sugar, cocoa butter, vanilla. Contains at least 70% cocoa.

Contains no additional additives. Has no negative impact on the microbiota.

70% dark chocolate Mild (Lindt) - cocoa mass, sugar, cocoa butter, emulsifier (SOY lecithin), vanilla. Contains at least 70% cocoa.

NOTE: the difference between the other 70% chocolate from Lindt, the mild variant contains emulsifiers.

If you want a chocolate bar without additives, choose regular 70% from Lindt.

PRINGLES ORIGINAL - VACUUM DRIED POTATOES, sunflower oil, wheat flour, corn flour, rice flour, maltodextrin, emulsifier (E471), salt, coloring (annatto extract norbixin).

PRINGLES SOUR CREAM & Onion - Vacuum dried potatoes, sunflower oil, wheat flour, corn flour, rice flour, sour cream and onion seasoning mix (wheat starch, flavor enhancer {monosodium glutamate, disodium guanylate, disodium inosinate}, onion powder, dextrose, sunflower oil, salt, modified corn starch, flavorings {milk}, maltodextrin, sugar, sweet whey powder {milk}, sour cream powder {milk}, glucose syrup powder, acids {citric acid, malic acid}, milk proteins), maltodextrin, emulsifier (E471), salt, coloring agent (annatto extract norbixin).

None of the Pringles products should be classified as food given that they do not contain real products but only processed products with additives. Sour cream & onion is full of additives that destroy your microbiota.

EXERCISE OR SEDENTARY BEHAVIOR

How much should you exercise to stay healthy and live long?

To be clear, exercise alone will not keep you healthy and allow you to grow old if you don't live a healthy lifestyle. For that to happen, you need to be a non-smoker, not drink too much alcohol, not stress, sleep poorly, be overweight or obese, you should eat a healthy and nutritional food and not eat and drink junk products.

ONE STUDY FOUND an association between exercise and a lower risk of all-cause mortality and cardiovascular disease.

The study also found that exercise does not reduce cardiovascular disease mortality and events in older adults or in people with chronic conditions.

This may be because there are underlying factors other than just exercise that affect how long we live.

. . .

A FINNISH STUDY from 2023 used data from more than 11 000 adult twins from the Finnish 'twin group'.

The amount of physical activity participants engaged in was assessed through questionnaires completed in 1975, 1981 and 1990. Participants were categorised into four groups: sedentary, moderately active, active and very active. Participants were followed for 45 years until 2020.

It was found that over a third - almost 40% - of the participants from the sedentary group had died during the follow-up up to 2020.

Participants in the active groups had between 15% and 23% lower risk of dying compared to the sedentary group.

The researchers then took into account other lifestyle factors, including body mass index (BMI), health status, alcohol use and smoking status.

When these factors are included, the mortality rate for participants in the sedentary group dropped to 7% i.e. the other factors contribute strongly to an increased mortality rate and reduce sedentariness as a single determinant of dying.

The researchers also found that participants in the sedentary and highly active groups both experienced accelerated biological aging compared to the moderately active and active groups.

IT IS HYPOTHESISED that the beneficial association of long-term exercise with reduced risk of death can be explained not only by exercise but also by other health-related factors.

Instead of regular physical activity being the cause of a lower risk of death, it may instead be an indicator of an overall healthy lifestyle, which helps to prolong a person's life. It is how we live our lives in general that affects our health outcomes.

MANY PEOPLE EXERCISE to gain health benefits, expecting it to offset unhealthy behaviors, which it does not.

Again, it is important to remember that physical activity does not outweigh an unhealthy diet, smoking, alcohol and drug use or other unhealthy activities, or ignoring high blood pressure, high cholesterol or diabetes.

A DANISH STUDY of patients with type 2 diabetes found that cycling reduced the risk of developing and dying from cardiovascular disease.

ANOTHER STUDY FOUND that you should walk 7 000 - 8 000 steps and then the benefits levelled off. So if you walk 20 000 steps a day, that's fine, but the health benefits compared to 7 000 steps do not increase.

EXERCISE AND DEMENTIA

One study measured the number of daily steps with pedometers in 78 000 people aged 40 to 79. It looked at total steps and whether the steps were insignificant ($<$40 steps/min), purposeful ($\geq$40 steps/min), and peak 30-minute intensity (average steps/min recorded for the highest, but not necessarily consecutive, 30 minutes of the day).

The number of people newly diagnosed with dementia was recorded 7 years later from medical and death records. After controlling for age, sex, ethnicity, education, socioeconomic status, smoking, alcohol, diet, medication, sleep, history of cardiovascular disease and days with a pedometer, the results showed that those who walked about 3 800 steps per day were 25% less likely to develop dementia, those who walked 9 800 steps per day had a 50% reduced risk of dementia, but additional steps did not increase the benefits.

It was seen that the greatest risk reduction for dementia was at around 6 300 vigorous steps per day (57% risk reduction) and at a 30-minute high-intensity walk of 112 steps/min (62% risk reduction).

In conclusion, the total number of steps in a day, and the intensity of those steps, matter in reducing the risk of dementia.

However, the minimum number of daily steps required to reduce the risk of dementia by 25% was only 3 800. A step count that is achievable for older people.

10 000 STEPS a day

It all started in 1965 when the Japanese company Yamasa Tokei began selling a new pedometer they called Manpo-kei ('ten thousand steps'). They combined the product launch with an advertising campaign - 'Let's walk 10 000 steps a day!' in an attempt to encourage physical activity. The recommendation was somewhat arbitrary, but from that point on, the 10 000 steps target was cemented in the public consciousness.

BUT WALKING FEWER steps still brings benefits. A study in JAMA followed a group of 2,100 people from the CARDIA study and found, unsurprisingly, that those with more steps per day had lower all-cause mortality. But interestingly, those who averaged 7 000 - 10 000 steps per day had as good an outcome as those who walked more than 10 000 steps, suggesting that the lower limit of 7 000 steps may be the desirable level.

An analysis of the US NHANES database showed less mortality for individuals who took more than 8 000 steps per day compared with those who took fewer than 4 000 steps. The benefits levelled out at 9 000-10 000 steps.

The point is that when it comes to physical activity, the biggest benefit seems to occur when you go from doing nothing to doing something.

Remember - you don't have to jog for it to be good for your health. Many people go from doing no exercise to trying to run 5 kilometres (3 miles). This is not a good tactic because there is a high risk that you will get injured, have severe exercise pain and then lose your motivation. If you are overweight, running puts a lot of strain on your feet, ankles, knees and hips.

Here's what to do:
Buy running shoes that are comfortable, have cushioning soles and good heel support. Start by walking at a slow pace for a few weeks. Then increase your walking pace for the next 3-4 weeks. After that, you can run 100 metres at a leisurely pace while walking to get your heart rate up.

Keep doing this and increase the distance and number of times you jog during your walk. Or walk on hilly terrain and at a brisk pace.

Exercise becomes more enjoyable when you realize the positive effects it has on your body and your health.

If you want to get your heart rate up and exercise in a gentle way - buy a bike.

Health is a lifelong behavior. You need to be patient because it takes time to establish new sustainable healthy habits.

SMOKING AND SNUS USE

E-cigarettes or vapes

Vapes are battery-powered products for inhaling smoke and have a container of 'e-liquid' made up of nicotine, propylene glycol, glycerol and flavorings such as banana, apple and cola. The liquid is heated and converted into vapour which is drawn into the lungs. Vapes cause respiratory problems in over 30% of users and in more than 50% of those who use both regular cigarettes and e-cigarettes. Ongoing Swedish research shows that e-cigarettes cause airway obstruction, inflammation, increased heart rate, higher blood pressure and stiffer blood vessels, i.e. the same health problems that regular cigarettes cause. Cell function is impaired and the risk of DNA damage increases.

(Heart and Lung Foundation, Sweden)

Tobacco smoking

Tobacco smoking has long been linked to cardiovascular disease and several cancers, not just lung cancer. There are over 7,000 studies showing the risks of smoking, so only recent findings are discussed here.

A STUDY from 2023 showed that smoking causes chromosomal damage in white blood cells which can accelerate the aging process.

In the analysis, based on almost half a million people, researchers reported that smokers were more likely to have shorter end fragments of chromosomes, known as 'telomeres' (usually likened to the plastic on the ends of shoelaces starting to unravel), which are well-known indicators of aging and of the ability of cells to repair and regenerate themselves.

Short telomeres were linked both to smoking and to the number of cigarettes smoked.

In other words, smoking can accelerate the aging process, while quitting smoking significantly reduces that process.

TOBACCO SMOKE IS TOXIC, and the cell damage it causes is not limited to visible symptoms like wrinkled skin. Cell damage occurs in all organs.

People who smoke many cigarettes had a significantly shorter telomere length, whereas in former smokers and never smokers this was not found.

Smoking is known to shorten life expectancy by an average of about 10 years.

PREMATURE AGING RELATED to chromosomal damage

means that even if you don't get cancer, premature aging will shorten your life.

In addition, premature aging can also affect your quality of life, including cognitive function, mobility, nutrition and social interaction.

Snus

Almost one in five men in Sweden use snus daily. Among women, 4% use snus. Snus also poses major health risks.

Nicotine is absorbed by the blood vessels in the oral mucosa and causes an immediate increase in blood pressure and heart rate. At the same time, it stresses the metabolism by increasing the secretion of adrenaline and other stress hormones. Studies show that snus has a detrimental effect on the inner walls of blood vessels, which is negative for cardiovascular health.

Anyone who snuff one snus-can a day or more increases their risk of developing type 2 diabetes by at least double.

According to Swedish studies, snus use by pregnant women is particularly problematic, with risks including miscarriage, pre-eclampsia, low birth weight, malformations and respiratory disorders. Snus use during pregnancy exposes the baby to nicotine levels as high as those seen in the mother. Nicotine can also be transferred to the baby during breastfeeding.

· · ·

AN INTERNATIONAL STUDY involving 9,000 people found that those who start to use snus before the age of 15 are at increased risk of developing asthma, especially among young women. The reason is believed to be the negative effects of snus on the lungs.

SOURCE: Heart and Lung Foundation, Sweden

21

———————

ALCOHOL

As with smoking, it is widely recognised that alcohol is harmful to us, especially if we drink often and if we drink too much. Harm and disease linked to alcohol seem to be directly proportional to the amount consumed.

ALCOHOL IS the cause of many accidents, violence and deaths. There is a high risk that we lose our judgement when we drink and make bad decisions as a result. Alcohol is high in calories and, because it is a poison, the body will always burn alcohol calories before calories from food and non-alcoholic drinks. This is why you gain weight more easily when drinking alcohol.

ON AVERAGE, we burn 0.1 grams of alcohol per kilogram of body weight per hour. It takes about two hours for a person weighing 60 kg (132 lb) to burn a standard glass of alcohol. A standard glass of alcohol contains 12 grams (0,4 oz) of pure alcohol. The combustion is linear, i.e. the same amount of alcohol is burnt every hour. It is therefore not possible to speed up the rate of combustion by, for example, going to the sauna, running, sleeping or using any medical preparation.

The metabolism takes place in the liver, which is often the first to be damaged and can lead to cirrhosis of the liver. Liver cancer often results if you continue to drink. But now there are also reports that colon cancer is linked to alcohol.

AWARENESS of the link between alcohol and cancer remains very low.

Almost half (46%) of the world's population consumes alcohol, and more men (54%) than women (38%).

Globally, the amount we drink averages around 6 litres (1,6 gallon) of pure alcohol per year per person, or about one bottle of wine per week.

However, consumption patterns vary widely from country to country. In France, people consume around 12 litres (3,2 gallon) per year or around two bottles of wine per week.

ALL ALCOHOL CONSUMPTION increases the risk of dementia, according to a new research. And it contradicts previous research that has suggested that light to moderate drinking can protect against dementia.

ALCOHOL IS a substance that has a depressant effect on the central nervous system, causing brain atrophy (the loss or reduction of brain cells). It is also a known neurotoxin (nerve poison). Alcohol can negatively affect the brain's memory centre, known as the hippocampus, by causing cell atrophy and by inhibiting the growth of new neurons via a process called neurogenesis. It is also known that chronic alcohol consumption can lead to a deficiency of an important B vitamin, thiamine, which is also very important for memory and cognition.

FOR MANY YEARS, it was thought that moderate alcohol intake could be beneficial for the heart, but more recent research contradicts this.

From a health perspective, there is no good reason to drink alcohol.

ACCORDING to data from the IARC (*International Agency for Research on Cancer*, the collaborating organization of the WHO and the United Nations that conducts and coordinates epidemiological research to combat cancer internationally), the following links between alcohol and cancer can be seen:

Heavy drinking - defined as more than 60 g/day or about 6 daily drinks - accounts for 47% of alcohol-related cancers.

Hazardous drinking - between 20 and 60 g/day or 2-6 daily drinks - accounts for 29%.

Moderate drinking - less than 20 g/day or about 2 daily drinks - accounts for about 14% of alcohol-related cancers.

Globally, alcohol accounted for 4% of all cancers diagnosed in 2020, according to IARC.

. . .

7 CANCER TYPES are linked to alcohol consumption - breast cancer, cancers of the oral cavity, pharynx, larynx, oesophagus, colorectal cancer and liver cancer, and emerging evidence suggests that cancers of the stomach and pancreas may also do so.

MALE POTENCY

An ever-present question is whether diet affects a man's potency. Many factors come into play, but diet is something that can be changed quite easily to improve potency.

ERECTILE DYSFUNCTION (IMPOTENCE), especially in younger men, is an early sign of cardiovascular disease and a cause of reduced quality of life.

ONE STUDY FOUND that men under 60 years of age who ate a Mediterranean diet had a lower risk of erectile dysfunction compared to men who did not follow the diet. The same favorable effect was also seen among older men, both in the 60 to 70 and over 70 age groups, who followed the Mediterranean diet.

· · ·

IN ANOTHER OBSERVATIONAL study of 250 middle-aged men with high blood pressure and erectile dysfunction, those who ate a Mediterranean diet had significantly higher testosterone levels, better exercise capacity and better erectile performance than those who did not eat the Mediterranean diet.

THIS IS likely because this dietary pattern may improve fitness and erectile performance by improving blood vessel function and limiting the decline in testosterone that occurs in middle age.

THE RESULTS SUGGEST that the Mediterranean diet may play an important role in maintaining several parameters of vascular health and quality of life in middle-aged men with hypertension and erectile dysfunction.

THE MEDITERRANEAN DIET also has a positive effect on the vessels of the heart and other important vessels in the body by improving the endothelial function of blood vessels (the function of blood vessel walls).

MICROPLASTICS

What are the health risks of microplastics?

The annual global production of plastics has increased exponentially from around 2 million tonnes in 1950 to 460 million tonnes in 2019, and current levels are expected to triple by 2060.

Plastics contain more than 10,000 chemicals, including carcinogens and endocrine disruptors. Plastics and their associated chemicals are responsible for pollution in the air, oceans, nature and the atmosphere.

The oceans are the ultimate destination for much of the plastic. All oceans, on the surface and in the depths, contain plastics, and there are even plastics in the polar ice caps.

Macro- and microplastic particles have been identified in hundreds of marine species, including the fish and shellfish we humans eat.

Food, drinks and food packaging emit micro- and nanoplastics. Water bottles represent a significant source of these plastics. About 90% are nanoplastics from packaging, which is two to three times more than previously estimated for microplastics.

We ingest micro- and nanoplastics when we eat and drink, when we breathe and through skin contact. For example, by drinking liquids or eating food that has been stored or heated in plastic containers that leak plastic particles. Or by using toothpaste containing micro- and nanoplastics.

A STUDY from September 2024 analysed the olfactory bulbs (upper nasal wall) of 15 deceased people and detected microplastics in the olfactory bulbs of 8 individuals. Plastic particles and fibres were found, with polypropylene being the most common plastic.

The presence of microplastics in the olfactory bulb area suggests that the olfactory pathway could be a potential entry point to the brain for microplastics with possible neurotoxic effects and implications for our health.

INFANTS ARE EXPOSED to micro- and nano-plastics from formula fed in polypropylene baby bottles, and at higher levels than previously thought, ranging from 14,600 to 4,550,000 particles per child per day.

STUDIES HAVE SHOWN that micro- and nanoplastics are a risk factor for cardiovascular disease and there is also a suspected link to inflammatory bowel disease, IBD (Crohn's disease, ulcerative colitis).

These plastic particles cause direct physical damage to, for example, the gut when we consume plastic-contaminated food, or the lungs when we breathe them in. The damage can then be caused by the plastic rubbing against the tissue.

Micro- and nano-plastics can also pose a chemical risk, as they contain other materials added during manufacturing to give them special properties such as strength, flexibility, stiffness, adaptability to external factors, etc.

Some of the most studied additives are phthalates and bisphenol A (BPA). Both are considered to be endocrine disruptors and can alter the functions of the endocrine system leading to adverse developmental, reproductive, neurological and even immune system effects.

Plastic particles can activate physical stress and cell damage, necrosis, inflammation, oxidative stress, and immune responses, which can contribute to the development of diseases such as cancer, metabolic disorders, and neuropsychiatric conditions, among others.

It has also been shown that plastics do not biodegrade easily, which means that once they enter the body, they can remain there for a very long time, posing a long-term health risk.

Processed and ultra-processed foods and beverages are more likely to contain these plastic particles.

The best advice is to be aware and avoid plastic products. Swap plastic bottles for metal or glass ones. Buy canned or glass bottled water instead of plastic bottles.

· · ·

MICROWAVE AND STORAGE

A study found that heating food in plastic containers in the microwave not only releases the microplastics, but also billions of nanoparticles and toxic chemicals from the plastic, which then end up in your food.

The study found that some packages released 4.2 million microplastics and 2.1 billion nanoplastic particles during 3 minutes in the microwave. It was also found that storing food in plastic packaging in the fridge and at room temperature for over six months released millions to billions of chemicals.

ADVICE: Do not microwave food in plastic packaging.

MICROPLASTICS in the carotid arteries

Patients with carotid stenosis (narrowing of the carotid artery) who were found to have microplastics in the stenosis had a higher risk of heart attack and stroke than people with carotid stenosis without plastic particles.

As previously described, we can inhale plastic particles or they can otherwise enter the bloodstream and further into the body tissue, and according to this study, it seems that nanoplastics have a tendency to settle in places where plaque deposition occurs more easily (carotid arteries, heart vessels) and cause inflammation.

In total, 58.4% of patients had a detectable amount of polyethylene (PE) in their plaques, and 12.1% had polyvinyl chloride (PVC).

After 34 months of follow-up, heart attack, stroke or death from any cause was found in 20% of patients with micro- or nanoplastics in their plaques, compared with 7.5% of those with carotid stenosis without plastic.

OTHER STUDIES HAVE FOUND plastic particles in the liver, placenta, breast milk, urine and blood.

24

CHEMICALS

The pandemic revealed an increasingly sick US population. Life expectancy dropped rapidly.

THREE QUARTERS of Americans are overweight or obese (and the situation is becoming quite comparable in Europe as well), half have diabetes or pre-diabetes, and a majority are metabolically unhealthy.

In addition, rates of allergic, inflammatory and autoimmune diseases are increasing by 3%-9% per year in the Western world.

Of course, diet and lifestyle are important factors behind this trend, but a vastly underestimated cause of illness is the role of environmental toxins and endocrine disrupting chemicals.

There is now growing evidence about their role in fertility, metabolic health and cancer. Although several toxic chemicals and toxins have been identified as carcinogens and legally regulated, many of them remain persistent in the environment and continue to be used.

Therefore, it is important to know who they are, how they harm us, so that we can avoid exposing ourselves to them.

HERE YOU CAN READ about some of the most common chemicals and the significant health risks associated with them, along with some general best practice advice on how to reduce the risk of exposure.

MICROPLASTICS - READ about these in the previous chapter.

PHTHALATES

Phthalates are chemicals used to make plastics softer and more durable, and to bind odours. They are commonly found in household items such as vinyl (e.g. floor mats, shower curtains) and fragrances, air fresheners and perfumes.

Phthalates are known endocrine disrupting chemicals, which when exposed have been associated with abnormal sex development and brain maturation in children, as well as lower levels of testosterone in men. Exposure is thought to occur through inhalation, ingestion and skin contact.

BISPHENOL A (BPA)

Bisphenol A is a chemical additive used to make clear and hard polycarbonate (PC) plastics, as well as epoxies (e.g. adhesives) and thermal paper (receipts).

Bisphenol A is one of the largest chemicals, with an

approximate annual production of 2.7 million tonnes. Bisphenol A is traditionally found in many clear plastic bottles and children's cups, but also on the inside of cans.

Structurally, Bisphenol A acts as a chemical that mimics the hormone oestrogen and has been associated with cardiovascular disease, obesity and male sexual dysfunction.

As with phthalates, the majority of what we ingest is believed to come from food products. In a study from the USA, Bisphenol A was found in more than 90% of participants.

Dioxins and polychlorinated biphenyls (PCBs)

Dioxins are mainly by-products of industrial manufacturing. They are released during combustion, when burning rubbish and in fires.

PCBs, which are somewhat structurally related to dioxins, were previously found in products such as flame retardants and refrigerants.

Dioxins have also been associated with a variety of health effects, impaired immunity and impacts on reproductive and endocrine systems.

High levels of PCB exposure have also been associated with an increased risk of mortality from cardiovascular disease.

Dioxin emissions have been reduced by 90% since the 1980s and PCBs have been banned from use in industrial manufacturing since 1979.

Dioxins are present in the environment and PCBs enter the food chain and are stored in fat.

The most effective ways to avoid exposure are to limit the consumption of meat, fish and dairy products and to remove the fat from meat.

The levels of dioxins and PCBs in meat, eggs, fish and dairy products are about 5-10 times higher than in plant-based foods.

Research has shown that farmed salmon is likely to be the most PCB-contaminated source of protein in the diet.

PESTICIDES

The rapid development of industrial agriculture over the last century has contributed to a dramatic increase in the use of industrial pesticides.

In fact, over 90% of the US population has pesticides in their urine and blood, regardless of where they live. The cause is thought to be food-related.

A LARGE EUROPEAN study showed a lower risk of cancer in people who consumed more organic food.

In addition, exposure to DDE - a metabolite of DDT, a chlorinated pesticide widely used in the 1940s and 1960s and still present in the environment today - has been shown to increase the risk of cognitive decline and Alzheimer's.

PER- AND POLYFLUORINATED ALKYL substances (PFAS)

PFAS are a group of fluorinated compounds discovered in the 1930s. Their chemical composition includes a durable carbon-fluoride bond, which means that they remain in the environment for thousands of years and are therefore known as 'forever chemicals'.

PFAS have been detected in the blood of 98% of Americans and in rainwater in places as far away as Tibet and

Antarctica. Even low levels of exposure have been associated with an increased risk of cancer, thyroid disease, birth defects, hormone disruption, reduced fertility and other serious health problems.

PFAS properties also make them durable at very high heat and they are also water repellent. For example, PFAS was used by 3M to make Scotchgard, a water repellent applied to fabric, furniture and carpets to protect them from stains, and by Dupont to make Teflon, a nonstick coating for pots and pans.

Although perfluorooctanoic acid (PFOA) was removed from nonstick cookware in 2013, PFAS - a family of thousands of synthetic compounds - is still common in fast food packaging, water- and stain-resistant clothing, personal hygiene products and firefighting foam. A group of people in Karlshamn, Sweden, sued the municipality, and won, for high levels of PFAS in drinking water caused by firefighting foam from the air force base in nearby town Kallinge. Among other things, an increase in the number of cancer cases among the residents was found.

You can search your municipality's website and see how much PFAS is in the drinking water. If this is not indicated, it may be a sign that the level is high and you should contact the municipality and ask for the PFAS level.

SOME PFAS also have surfactant properties that make them useful in cleaning products, floor polish, car care products, paint, ski wax and cosmetics (make-up, sun cream, skin cream, foundation cream).

Less known uses of PFAS are in dental materials, medical devices, dirt repellents for building materials, smartphones and solar cells.

PFAS are released into the environment during the degradation of these products, as well as when dumped from waste facilities.

BENZOPHENONE, which is strongly suspected of being carcinogenic, is used in cosmetics, sunscreens, moisturisers, shampoos, hair care products, cosmetics (lipsticks, lip balms, creams and lotions), nail varnishes, plastics and dental composite materials.

25

STRESS, NOISE AND SLEEP

Stress is, from an evolutionary perspective, a reaction that occurs in the body when we are exposed to danger. A number of hormones are released (adrenaline, noradrenaline and cortisol) and put us on alert for flight or fight. Today, it is rare for those of us living in the Western world to need to flee or fight. However, other events can trigger the activation of stress hormones, and when we live with a constant build-up of stress hormones, it can lead to diseases.

ONE STUDY (NEURON) showed that the combination of stress and comfort eating switches off the brain's mechanism that tells you when you have eaten enough (blocks the feeling of fullness).

This can lead to overeating when comfort eating, with the consequence that it leads to weight gain and obesity, which in turn can lead to even more stress.

• • •

Research from Germany (Circulation Research) shows that noise has harmful effects on the heart and blood vessels.

Noise from road, rail or air traffic increases the risk of cardiovascular morbidity such as ischaemic heart disease, heart failure, stroke, and increased risk of mortality. Traffic noise at night leads to disturbed sleep with awakening and shortened sleep, an increase in stress hormones and increased oxidative stress in the vessels and in the brain, and to inflammation, high blood pressure and thus increased cardiovascular risk.

Noise also puts the body on alert and activates the autonomic nervous system, releasing the stress hormones adrenaline and cortisol, leading to an increase in heart rate and blood pressure.

According to the study, people perceive aircraft noise as the most annoying, followed by road, neighbourhood, industrial and railway noise.

Another study (JAMA) found that sleep duration and sleep patterns of short or unstable sleep were significantly associated with an increased risk of cardiovascular disease and mortality.

People who reported always sleeping less than 5 hours per night had the highest risk of both cardiovascular disease and death.

One study (JAMA) has also found associations between sleep duration and cognitive impairment, both in people with insufficient sleep ($\leq$4 hours per night) but also in those who slept too much ($\geq$10 hours per night).

. . .

A STUDY in Nature Communications found an increased risk of dementia in people who sleep less than 6 hours a night in their 50s and 60s compared to those who sleep at least 7 hours each night.

There is also strong evidence that sleep becomes abnormal before dementia is diagnosed. However, this still does not explain whether it is poor sleep that triggers dementia or makes it worse, as the changes in the brain that cause dementia start many years before dementia is diagnosed. It is known that advanced dementia is associated with poor sleep.

ANOTHER STUDY (SLEEP and Breathing) suggests that certain unhealthy sleep behaviors are associated with an increased risk of leading to fewer healthy years of life.

The researchers looked at the association between four sleep behaviors: difficulty falling asleep/insomnia, napping, daytime sleepiness and difficulty getting out of bed, and whether this occurred 'often' or 'rarely/never', and then linked it to diseases and fewer healthy years.

Fewer years of health were defined by eight conditions - heart failure, heart attack, chronic obstructive pulmonary disease (COPD), stroke, dementia, diabetes, cancer and death.

People who 'frequently had difficulty falling asleep or experienced insomnia', 'frequently took a nap', 'frequently felt excessively sleepy during the day' and who had 'difficulty getting out of bed' had an increased risk of having fewer healthy years of life.

. . .

A STUDY (JOURNAL of the American College of Cardiology) of sleep-deprived young adults linked sleep deprivation to abdominal obesity and to harmful visceral fat or 'belly fat'.

People who were sleep deprived ate an average of 308 calories more per day than the group who slept longer, leading to a 0.5 kg weight gain after two weeks, but it also led to an increase of 7,8 m^2 of tissue fat around the intestines, equivalent to an increase of around 11%.

After a recovery period, it was found that visceral adipose tissue in the sleep-deprived subjects continued to increase, even though body weight dropped and subcutaneous fat decreased. Although the subjects slept longer, ate fewer calories and lost weight, their abdominal fat continued to increase, gaining an additional 3.125 m^2 on average by day 21.

IN ANOTHER STUDY (CLINICAL NUTRITION), researchers examined the dietary intake and perceived stress of over 8,600 Australians aged 25 years and older and found that those with the highest intake of fruit and vegetables had 10% lower scores of 'perceived stress' compared to the lowest intake of fruit and vegetables. The association was strongest in middle-aged people compared to younger people or those of retirement age.

Bioactive nutrients and phytochemicals including vitamins C, E, K and B group vitamins, carotene and phenolic compounds found in fruit and vegetables may play a role in reducing stress levels.

When analysing whether there were gender differences, it was found that a high intake of fruit and vegetables was associated with lower perceived stress in both genders.

. . .

How LACK of sleep is reflected in our blood markers

Our need for sleep varies from person to person, but most adults need between seven and eight hours a night to feel good. Sleeping less than six hours per night for an extended period of time increases the risk of infections, metabolic diseases and cardiovascular problems.

HERE ARE some of the markers most affected by lack of sleep.

1. Elevated inflammation markers

Lack of sleep is strongly linked to increased inflammation in the body. In case of prolonged lack of sleep, the inflammation marker C-reactive protein (CRP) increases, which signals that the body is stressed. Elevated inflammation, in turn, has been linked to cardiovascular and metabolic diseases, making CRP an important indicator to monitor.

Blood test: hs-CRP (high-sensitivity CRP)

2. Elevated blood sugar and insulin levels

Sleep is also crucial to keeping blood sugar levels stable. With a lack of sleep, insulin's ability to regulate glucose is impaired, which leads to higher blood sugar levels and can develop into insulin resistance – a risk factor for type 2 diabetes. In blood tests, this shows up as elevated glucose values and altered insulin sensitivity, which increases the risk of diabetes and other metabolic diseases.

Blood test: C-peptide, HbA1C, Glucose

3. Elevated cortisol levels

Cortisol is a hormone that helps the body deal with stress and regulates important functions such as blood pressure and blood sugar. Normally, cortisol levels are highest in the morning and decrease throughout the day. With a lack of sleep, cortisol levels can remain high even in the evening, which disrupts the body's circadian rhythm. Elevated cortisol levels are a sign of chronic stress, which in the long run negatively affects the immune system and heart health.

Blood test: Cortisol

4. Changes in the immune system

Sleep is critical for the immune system. With a lack of sleep, the amount of white blood cells decreases, especially so-called natural killer cells (NK cells), which protect the body against viruses and bacteria. With prolonged lack of sleep, the levels of these cells drop, making the body more vulnerable to infections.

Blood test: LPK (leukocytes), lymphocytes

5. Elevated blood lipids

Long-term lack of sleep can also affect blood fats, including triglycerides and LDL cholesterol, the "bad" cholesterol. Studies have shown that lack of sleep can lead to an increased appetite for fatty and sweet foods, which affects blood lipids and contributes to an increased risk of cardiovascular disease.

Blood tests: Triglycerides, LDL cholesterol

THIS IS how you can improve your sleep quality

Make sure you get a good dose of daylight in the morning hours as it resets our biological clock. When the morning light hits the eye, signals are sent to our brain (including the pineal gland) and the body's rhythm is synchronized with the time of day. Try to be outside for 20 minutes, even if it's cloudy, or sit near a window.

Keep it cool in the bedroom (about 18 degrees). You can also take a warm shower before bedtime.

Reduce the lighting in the evening, when the production of the body's sleep hormone melatonin is initiated.

It should be dark in the bedroom. When it's dark, your body senses that it's time to sleep, which secretes the sleep hormone melatonin.

Install a blackout roller blind or equivalent. Use a blindfold if you cannot darken the bedroom. If you often sleep in hotels and have problems with sleep, bring a blindfold and earplugs.

Avoid screens with blue light 2 hours before bedtime. The blue light interferes with the production of melatonin.

Unwind before bed.

Go to bed at the same time every night. The body likes routines!

Avoid alcohol or drink in moderation as alcohol disrupts sleep.

Review your nutritional intake. Deficiencies in vitamin D, vitamin B12, vitamin E, vitamin B6 and C have been linked to impaired sleep and sleep apnea.

Try to schedule your workout early in the day instead of in the evening. Being active and going out too much in the evening can raise cortisol levels just as you are about to fall asleep.

Do not drink coffee or tea or after lunch. Never drink energy drinks. These drinks also destroy your microbiota.

Do not eat dinner too close to bedtime, it can be difficult to fall asleep when digestion is in full swing.

Sleeping in on the weekends may actually be good, according to new reports.

Don't drink late at night because then the risk of waking up and having to go to the toilet increases. If you have difficulty falling asleep when you wake up during the night, it is even more important not to drink late at night.

Use earplugs if you wake up easily or are disturbed by noise.

If you live in a noisy environment, if possible, change to another bedroom without disturbing noise.

26

TIPS ON EXERCISE

Here are some tips on how to move your body during the day. Personally, I hate when my body goes limp and find that where I once had muscle, there is now just skin and fat. That is why I have introduced these daily exercises. And remember, for the exercises to be done, you need to build up a daily routine and not deviate from it. You must have self-discipline! If you start skipping the exercises, the lazy routine will quickly take over.

Squat

If you have a sedentary job, this is an easy way to activate your leg muscles while releasing many beneficial substances into your body. As we get older, we lose muscle mass and this makes us weaker and impairs our balance. Squats build thigh muscles and glutes. Adopting this routine can reduce the risk of falls and injuries as we get older.

20-30 squats every one or two hours (or as many as you can manage).

. . .

Push-ups

Every morning after breakfast I do push-ups. Since it puts a little strain on the shoulders, it is recommended not to go deeper than 90 degrees, that is, the elbows are at a right angle when you are at your deepest. For me, sometimes it can take 15-30 minutes between sets, but the most important thing is that you do them.

40 push-ups x 3 (or as many as you can do)

Arms and shoulders

I have a rubber band with a handle, model Refit (Google). I have tested a few different products, but Refit is the rubber band that has been the most durable so far.

Every weekday I train biceps, triceps and shoulders. Not to become a bodybuilder, but to maintain muscle mass.

Biceps: Do as many biceps curls as you can handle x 3. I place my feet on the rubber band and can thus vary how heavy it gets.

Triceps: Standing triceps curl behind the back x 3.

Shoulders: Standing arm lift to the sides x 3.

Walk - bike

During spring, summer and autumn I usually cycle as exercise. I think it puts less strain on the joints and you can exert yourself more without getting as tired as when you jog. I can also recommend cycling as a holiday. You get to experience and see a lot and you invest in your health and get fitness in the bargain.

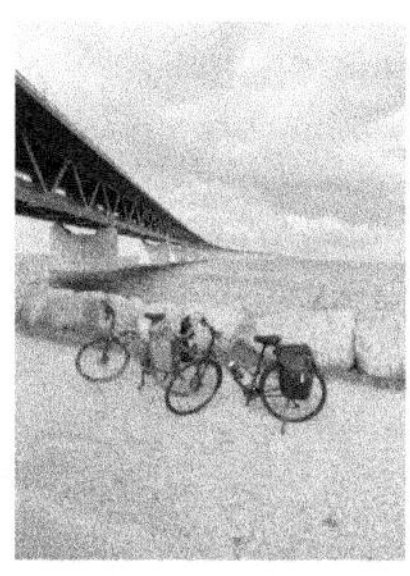

My favorite bridge, Öresundsbron, between Sweden and Denmark (2023)

But how you exercise and what type of exercise you prefer is individual. **The important thing is THAT you exercise.**

A SIMPLE FORM of exercise that almost everyone can do is walking. Science has concluded that 7,000 to 10,000 steps a day at a brisk, fast pace, preferably in hilly terrain, is the amount that best benefits your health. If you walk more, that's fine, but it has not been shown to improve health further. You can also break up your walks throughout the day.

SUPPLEMENTS - WHICH ONES SHOULD YOU TAKE

Probiotics
The good bacteria that we feed our gut microbiota are called probiotics. If we eat a lot of fibre, which is found in vegetables, fruit, legumes, whole grains etc, we provide food and energy to the gut bacteria. When they get fibre, the good bacteria increase in diversity, ie both the number of bacteria and bacterial strains.

You can also add good bacteria to your gut by eating fermented foods such as fermented vegetables (read the chapter on 'Fermentation'), sauerkraut (don't buy sauerkraut that has been pasteurized because the good bacteria die in that process), kimchi, kefir, kombucha, sourdough bread (be aware that many breads you buy in the grocery stores contains far too little sourdough) or by taking probiotic supplements.

There are probiotics supplement that contains only one bacteria strain and others that contain many strains. Most supplements contain up to 10 billion bacteria.

Be aware that the Western diet is low in fibre. Meat is

also low in fibre and the ultra-processed foods and drinks (soft drinks, energy drinks) that many people consume on a daily basis destroy the microbiota, leading to a dysbiosis. Because of that, there is a great need for many people to take probiotics. Just remember that if you take probiotics and at the same time eat and drink ultra-processed products, you will destroy diversity of the microbiota that you are building up.

Recommendation

Eat fruits, vegetables, legumes and whole grains. Ferment yourself as it is very easy to do.

Take supplements and choose a product that contains 5-8 different strains of bacteria, preferably Bifidobacterium lactis and Lactobacillus rhamnosus as these are the most studied.

SELENIUM

Selenium is an element found in soil. Selenium is part of enzymes that protect cells from oxidation, interacts with vitamin E and participates in immunological defense mechanisms.

Selenium is found in almost all foods, but levels vary. In some countries, the soil is poor in selenium, so vegetables grown there have a low content of selenium. The foods that contain the most selenium are fish, shellfish, offal, nuts/seeds such as Brazil nuts and sunflower seeds, lentils, eggs and cheese.

Severe selenium deficiency can lead to heart muscle changes, for example, but selenium deficiency is rare. There are studies indicating that insufficient selenium is associated with an increased risk of certain cancers.

According to the Swedish National Food Agency, the

daily intake should not exceed 255 micrograms (0.000009 oz).

Q10

Coenzyme Q10 is a vitamin-like substance with antioxidant properties that is found throughout the body's cells. Coenzyme Q10 is a substance needed for the body's cells to produce energy.

The amount of Q10 in tissues decreases in older people and with a sedentary lifestyle. Q10 is found in red meat, oily fish, chicken, rapeseed oil, walnuts, peanuts, sesame seeds, pistachios, broccoli and cauliflower. However, most of the body's Q10 is made by the body itself. The diet provides only small amounts.

A Swedish-Norwegian study (BMC Medicine) investigated the effect of the combination of selenium and Q10 on older people and found that the combination may have beneficial effects on thyroid hormones, that it reduces cardiovascular mortality and increases quality of life in people with insufficient thyroid function due to selenium and Q10 deficiency.

Recommendation

Elderly people lose the ability to produce Q10 and therefore its supplementation in combination with Selenium may be recommended.

Magnesium

Magnesium is needed, among other things, for the production of protein, for the metabolism of calcium and for normal nerve and muscle function.

Magnesium is mainly found in legumes, leafy vegetables, whole grain products and meat, fish and seafood. We also get magnesium through the water we drink, especially in municipalities with hard water.

Magnesium deficiency can lead to stunted growth, behavioral problems and cardiac dysfunction. Severe magnesium deficiency can cause seizures.

An upper limit for safe intake of magnesium from food supplements is set at 250 mg per day according to the Swedish National Food Agency.

Recommendation

Take magnesium supplements if your drinking water is soft and if you are prone to cramps. Should be taken in the evening.

Vitamin D

Vitamin D is needed to build strong teeth and bones. Vitamin D is one of the few vitamins we risk getting too little of.

We get vitamin D in two ways: firstly, through food, and secondly, vitamin D is formed in the skin when we are out in the sun. We get most of our vitamin D from food when we eat oily fish. Oily fish, such as salmon, herring and mackerel, are high in vitamin D. In many countries most dairy products, plant-based drinks, sandwich fats and spreads are fortified with vitamin D. These fortified foods are important sources of vitamin D.

Recommendation

Take vitamin D supplements. However, there is disagreement about how much vitamin D we need to take as a supplement. The maximum dose is 100 mg per day. 75 mg corresponds to 3000 IU and is a common dose in supplement products.

. . .

Zinc

Zinc is a vital mineral. Zinc is part of 100s of enzymes in the body that affect the metabolism of proteins, carbohydrates, fats, nucleic acids (chemical compounds that occur naturally in living organisms in the form of DNA and RNA) and certain vitamins such as vitamin A.

Zinc is also needed for the immune system. Meat, dairy products, whole grain products, mussels, cheese and nuts are rich in zinc. The risk of zinc deficiency is low.

Recommendation

You probably do not need to take extra zinc supplements if you eat a healthy diet. Eat pecans, cashews and peanuts if you want to get extra zinc. Remember that nuts should be natural without extra salt and fat and that nuts are high in calories.

HEALTH EXAMINATION

A health check is a way of getting feedback on how good your health is. Many companies offer health checks to their employees, so start by checking if your company offer that.

IF YOU WANT to lose weight, you need to know how much you weigh before you start losing weight, what your target weight is and whether you are losing weight as planned.

Similarly, you should know your health status before you start your change. How are your health values today compared to when you reach your goal? When you get your results back and your health parameters are outside the reference values, you should consult your doctor.

THE FOLLOWING TESTS ARE RECOMMENDED.

ECG

An ECG shows how fast your heart beats, certain heart diseases, congenital heart defects, current or previous heart attacks, myocardial inflammation, thickening of the heart muscle and disturbances of the heart rhythm, such as atrial fibrillation.

Exercise ECG (Stress test)

An exercise ECG test how your heart, lungs, blood circulation and musculoskeletal system works when you exert yourself. The purpose is to find out if the heart is getting enough oxygen and if you experience chest pain or arrhythmia during exercise. Clogged vessels may show up as a reduced oxygenation of the heart and as a disturbance in the ECG curve.

Lab test of your blood

(tests can probably also be purchased at private labs)

Cardiovascular markers

- Total cholesterol
- LDL cholesterol
- HDL cholesterol
- non-HDL cholesterol
- Triglycerides
- Lipoprotein (a)

Blood sugar test

- HbA1c (called 'long-term sugar' and indicates risk of type 2 diabetes)

BLOOD AND IRON

- Haemoglobin
- Leucocytes
- Erythrocytes
- Platelets

VITAMINS

- Vitamin B12
- Folate

INFLAMMATION

- hs-CRP (high-sensitivity C-reactive protein, NOTE not the ordinary test for infection)

THYROID GLAND

- TSH (thyroid stimulating hormone)

LIVER

- AST
- ALT

KIDNEYS

- Calcium
- Potassium
- Sodium
- Creatinine
- eGFR

FOR men

- PSA (Prostate-Specific Antigen - a test for prostate cancer)

IF YOU ARE over 50 years old (men and women)

- Stool sample to test for colorectal cancer

FERMENTATION - RECIPES

Fermenting vegetables

Fermenting vegetables is very easy and delicious.

Start by buying one or more glass jars with a rubber gasket and locking device. It is necessary because the liquid vegetables will ferment and leak.

INGREDIENTS

Decide vegetables. Suggestions are white cabbage, pointed cabbage or savoy cabbage, carrots, radishes, cauliflower, broccoli, onions, leeks, courgettes, ginger, garlic, chilli. Use salt without iodine to stir into water.

My favourites are savoy cabbage, carrots, cauliflower, onion, ginger, chilli, garlic.

INSTRUCTION

1. Cut the vegetables into bite-sized pieces. When you've sliced them, put them in a larger bowl so

    you can mix them around before you press them into the jar.

2. Add the vegetables to the jar and squeeze well.
3. Pour 1 litre of cold water into a large bowl and 1 tablespoon of salt WITHOUT iodine (iodine hinders the fermentation process). Stir until the salt is dissolved.
4. Pour the liquid into the jar until it reaches 0.5-1 cm from the edge. Personally, I usually make several jars at once and then more liquid is needed.
5. Place the jar(s) in a dish with a slightly higher rim, as liquid will sip out when the fermentation process starts. There will also be a slight odour of yeast but this will disappear after a couple of days.
6. Leave the jar(s) at room temperature for 2 weeks. Not in direct sunlight.
7. After 2 weeks, put the jars in the fridge for another 2 weeks, then they are ready to eat. They now contain lots of probiotics (the good bacteria) which can help improve the diversity of the microbiota.
8. Eat some every evening with dinner.

FERMENTATION LASTS for several months when stored in the refrigerator.

KIMCHI

    Kimchi is a little more laborious to make but on the

other hand, it gets ready faster. You can choose to make a vegan version and then you just exclude the seafood ingredients. Personally, I think it tastes just as good without them.

You will need the same jars as described in fermentation.

INGREDIENTS

1.5 - 2kg of salad cabbage

3.5 - 4 tablespoons of salt without iodine (1 tablespoon per pint of water)

1.5 - 2 litres of water

2 tbsp rice flour

1 tbsp granulated sugar

2-3 tbsp grated ginger

5 pcs garlic, grated

1 coarsely grated yellow onion

1 1/4 dl fish sauce (can be omitted if you want it completely plant-based)

1 dl gochugaru (if you don't want it too strong, just use a little less than a dl)

6 thinly sliced spring onions

Carrots, 3-4 pieces, thinly sliced

10 cm thinly sliced radishes in rods

Apple, 2 pcs, tart and firm. Cut into 0.5 cm thin sticks.

1 dl light soya sauce

INSTRUCTIONS

1. Peel and rinse the salad bowl. Cut the lettuce into 4 cm pieces and place in a large bowl. Separate the leaves well. Sprinkle with the salt and mix gently but thoroughly to cover all the leaves with salt. Leave to stand for 1.5 hours.
2. An alternative way, which I prefer instead of salting and mixing, is to stir the salt into water and pour it over so that the water covers the cabbage. Leave to stand for 1.5 hours.
3. Pour off the salt water and rinse the cabbage thoroughly to remove excess salt. Feel free to flavor the cabbage so that it has the right saltiness.
4. Pour the water, rice flour and sugar into a saucepan and boil to a thick liquid sauce. Leave to cool slightly by placing the pan in cold water. Then mix in the ginger, garlic, onion, fish sauce (or exclude for plant-based option) and gochugaru. Add the spring onion, carrot, radish, apple to the salad bowl and pour over the sauce and mix thoroughly.

TRANSFER TO GLASS JARS, press down and close the lid. Don't fill the jars to the top, but leave a couple of cm, you need space for the fermentation process. Leave at room temperature for 2-3 days, preferably with plastic bags over the lids, as liquid may splash out when fermentation starts. Then store in the refrigerator. Best after 2 weeks but kimchi will keep for at least 3 months. After 3-4 weeks, the fermented flavor that kimchi gives off when it is most lactic acidified disappears.

30

SOURDOUGH, BREAD, MUESLI - RECIPES

I n this chapter you will find recipes on how to start a sourdough starter and how to keep it alive, how to make a tasty and healthy bread and how to easily make your own muesli.

SOURDOUGH

All you need is flour, and water. Bread baked with sourdough is extra tasty and it's also good for your microbiota, and therefore good for your whole body.

SOURDOUGH CAN BE MADE with any flour that contains gluten. I prefer whole grain flour as I feel that it provides better fermentation capacity and it is easier to get the sourdough started.

THE TYPE of flour I have chosen is dinkel (spelt) whole grain flour and I find that it is easy to keep going and works

181

well in bread baking. And it has stayed alive for 3.5 years without any problems.

I use organic flour because that type of flour contains more of the good bacteria that the microbiota wants.

How to do it:

Get a glass jar (volume about 10 dl), preferably one with a metal lock over a hook. But you should remove the rubber gasket from the lid, so that it does not become too tight.

Do this on days 1 - 3
Ingredients
1.5 dl whole grain flour
1 dl room temperature water

Instructions for use

Day 1

1. Mix 1 dl room temperature water with 1.5 dl whole grain flour in the glass jar and close the lid, but not so tightly. Air must be able to get in, but not bugs.
2. Stir until it becomes a thicker pancake batter.
3. Store the jar at room temperature. Not in direct sunlight.

. . .

DAY 2

1. Some small bubbles may have formed in the batter, but don't panic if they haven't. Sometimes it takes longer. The batter may also have a fresh and aromatic flavor now.
2. Now add the same amount of flour and water as Day 1, stir and close the lid.
3. Keep the jar in the same place.

DAY 3

1. Add the same amount of flour and water one last time.
2. Store the jar in the same place.

DAY 4

1. By now, your sourdough should be ready to be used in baking and you should see more bubbles than yesterday. It should also smell a little sour.
2. If there are too few bubbles or if it doesn't smell sour, you can repeat the procedure for another day.

THE LID of the jar should be slightly ajar, especially at the beginning. This allows the bacteria and oxygen in the air to get in and get the sourdough going. However, the lid should not be completely open, because then you risk getting unwanted bugs etc. The sourdough also risks drying out.

IF IT TAKES a long time for the sourdough to get going, it may be due to several different things, including the room temperature. If the room is too cold, it may take a little longer.

When the sourdough is ready, store it in the fridge.

FEED the sourdough

Feed it about once a week. To do this, stir 1 tbsp of dinkel flour and just under 1 tbsp of cold water into the sourdough. Then put it back in the fridge.

BEFORE BAKING

BEFORE YOU BAKE, start a larger volume of sourdough.

24 HOURS before you will bake add 1 dl of dinkel flour and just under 1 dl of cold water to the sourdough, then put it back in the fridge.

RECIPES FOR BREAD

I have experimented with several different types of

flour. You can vary the flours as needed to make different types of bread. Remember that the more weight of gluten in the flour, the easier the dough will fall apart.

Use organic flour.

Do this 10-12 hours before baking the dough.

INGREDIENTS:

50 grams sifted dinkel flour

250 grams of whole grain dinkel (ancient wheat flour)

250 grams of Einkorn whole grain (oldest wheat flour)

250 grams of whole grain naked barley (old barley flour)

18 grams of salt (NB without iodine, otherwise the leavening process may stop)

8-10 grams of yeast

150 grams of sourdough

5 dl water (lukewarm)

Option 1: 1 jar of pitted olives (250-300 grams of pitted olives)

Option 2: 300 grams of walnuts

Scale that measures in grams

DO IT LIKE THIS:

It helps a lot if you have a scale with a 1 gram setting, which you can reset once the bowl is placed on the scale and after each new type of flour you weigh.

PLACE the bowl on the scale, zero it and pour in the flour.

Zero the scales after each new type of flour you add. In total, there should be about 800 grams of flour.

Take a small bowl and weigh out 18 grams of salt and stir into the flour.

Pour 5 dl of water into a saucepan and heat until lukewarm. Add the yeast and sourdough and whisk until it dissolves in the water. Pour the liquid into the flour and work until it becomes a fine dough. Add the drained olives or walnuts and stir into the dough.

Take out a new bowl/bowl to hold the dough, pour in some olive oil and grease the edges of the bowl so that the dough will release more easily once it has finished rising.

Cover the bowl and place in the fridge for 10-12 hours.

Take the bowl out of the fridge about 1 hour before putting the dough in the oven.

Preheat the oven to 200 degrees (over/under heat).

Pour the dough onto a baking tray greased with olive oil to make it easier to work. Shape the dough into an oblong and fairly long shape.

· · ·

ONCE YOU HAVE SHAPED the dough, place the tray in the oven immediately. After 15 minutes, reduce the temperature to 150°C and leave the dough to bake for another 1.5 hours.

TAKE THE DOUGH OUT. Place it on a wooden cutting board (never use a plastic cutting board if you want to avoid ingesting plastic) and leave it to cool under a towel.

You can cut the bread into slices once it has cooled and store in the freezer (in paper bags, avoid plastic bags).

Take a slice of bread and toast it for breakfast. Nutritious and delicious.

MUESLI

The choice of ingredients is optional. Here is a suggested recipe.

1500 GR OF OATS, spelt, rye, emmer wheat, barley, naked oats (choose according to variety)

500 gr of walnuts

200 hazelnuts

200 gr cashew

200 gr sunflower seeds

(200 gr pumpkin seeds if the price is not too high)

HOW TO DO IT:

1. put the oven on 150 degrees hot air

2. Pour the cereal mixture into a long pan with high sides. Make sure the flakes are evenly distributed.

3. Put the tray in the oven for 20 minutes. Take out and stir.

4. Put the tray back in and repeat step 3. The procedure is then repeated once more.

5. When the tray has been in 3 times, pour over the nuts and seeds and mix with the flakes.

6. Put the tin in for a final 20 minutes. Check that the nuts are not burnt.

SUMMARY - AN EASY TRANSITION TO A HEALTHIER LIFE

How do you want your retirement life to be like? Many people plan to spend more time with their children and grandchildren. They plan to do and experience things they never had the chance to do before.

But to be able to do all that, you need to be a healthy retiree, and to be one, you need to invest in your health. And the earlier you start, the better returns you will get. It's as obvious as if you don't service and look after your car, it will stop working prematurely.

THERE ARE two details in particular that are especially important if you want to be healthy and live a long life - building diversity in your gut microbiota and eating an anti-inflammatory diet.

IF YOU FOLLOW these simple tips on what to eat more of, what to eat less of, and what to avoid altogether, you'll be well on your way to becoming a healthy, long-lived person.

But it is also scientifically established that the younger you are when you start your change, the more healthy years you will have. But it's never too late to start gaining healthy years.

It is always what is easy to accomplish that becomes successful, therefore becoming healthier must be easy. But a change is not very meaningful if it is not sustainable in the long run.

To change your lifestyle in an easy way, start by adding fruit, vegetables, pulses, whole-grains, to your meals and cut down on high fat and sugar foods and completely remove ultra-processed foods and drinks.

Add and remove one thing at a time. Taste will determine the success of your transition, so don't forget to season your food. However, be careful with the salt.

This will be easy for you. You can choose freely from the list below and add whatever you feel like. The gut bacteria want a variety of fibre for everyone to get theirs, so feel free to vary what you eat a lot of.

Eat plenty of

Fruit, vegetables, leafy greens (rocket, spinach), root vegetables, legumes (lentils, beans), whole grains (muesli, bread baked with whole grain flour), nuts (especially walnuts and pecans), seeds (sunflower seeds, pumpkin seeds), fermented products (NB not pasteurised because the good bacteria die in the process - sauerkraut is often pasteurised), sprouts (it's easy to sprout alfalfa seeds and mung beans)

EAT LESS of

Red meat (beef, pork), fish, shellfish, chicken, alcohol, salt.

Do you want to eat meat? Be aware that there is a reason why the Nordic Nutrition Recommendations limit the amount to 350 grams per week. If you eat meat, eat pasture-raised animals and not industrially raised ones.

Do you want to eat fish? Avoid farmed fish as they are raised on concentrated feed and medicines to grow fast and to avoid diseases and parasites common in the ponds where 10,000s of fish are crowded.

You should also take into account that the oceans are increasingly polluted by microplastics. These plastics end up in fish and shellfish and then in you when you eat.

IN THE CHICKEN and egg industries, many animals are crowded together. Salmonella outbreaks are not uncommon, with entire flocks of 100,000s of chickens or hens being culled. Campylobacter is another common bacteria you can contract if the chicken is undercooked.

In USA the food organisation has accepted that 25% of

chicken bought in the grocery store can be infected with salmonella. It's up to consumers to cook in correct way to kill the bacterias.

Dairy products such as cheese, yoghurt (sweetened with sugar or sweeteners). If you want yoghurt, choose kefir which is fermented and good for your stomach.

Never eat or drink

Processed and ultra-processed foods (the more ingredients, the more ultra-processed) such as sausages, charcuterie, liver pate, industrially produced foods such as frozen pizza, deep-fried chicken nuggets, white bread, industrially baked bread, cakes, soups, sweets, ice cream, crisps, soft drinks (both with sugar and artificial sweeteners), energy drinks (both with sugar and artificial sweeteners), farmed fish.

Intermittent fasting - time-restricted eating

Fasting has long been recognised as healthy. The 5:2 diet, where you eat for 5 days and fast for 2 days, became a popular method pioneered by Michael Mosley.

More recently, other types of fasting have become popular and are called intermittent fasting or Time Restricted Eating (TRE).

This involves having so-called eating windows, which is a period during the day when you eat your meals for the day and fast the rest of the time. A window of 6-10 hours is common. However, you must drink, preferably water. Coffee or tea is also fine, but not in large quantities.

VARIATIONS OF TIME-RESTRICTED EATING:
Eat breakfast and lunch but not dinner.
Lunch and dinner but not breakfast.
Breakfast and dinner but not lunch.
I use the last variant and instead of eating lunch I exercise.

IT CAN TAKE a few days for your body to adjust to not getting food and during those days you will be a little hungry. But once your body has adjusted, you won't feel hungry. Your blood sugar will be more stable because your body has realized that it will not be fed and therefore does not need to secrete insulin to remove the sugar from your bloodstream.

In comparison, when you eat at regular intervals, your body becomes attuned to frequent meals and signals with feelings of hunger - that now is the time to eat.

OTHER BENEFITS of time-restricted eating are that you lose weight or find it easier to maintain your weight. Fasting has a positive effect on the cells involved in the aging process, and the vast majority of researchers on aging use time-restricted eating.

It also has a positive effect on inflammation in the body, partly because of its effect on aging cells, but also because it is beneficial for the gut microbiota.

Scientists have explained that even the gut bacteria

need to rest and not work all the time. And based on that hypothesis, it should be best to skip lunch. This gives the gut bacteria two longer periods of rest.

Fasting keeps blood sugar levels stable.

Be aware of

It takes about 20 minutes for satiety signals to reach the brain, so eat slowly.

Vegetables are filling, high in fibre and low in calories. Therefore you can eat more of these.

Do not eat late at night. And at least 3 hours before going to bed.

Fermentation

Fermentation is an ancient preservation method. Vegetables are left to ferment, which causes bacteria to grow and produce lactic acid and carbon dioxide as they break down carbohydrates.

Fermented vegetables contain not only the fibre and nutrients that the gut bacteria feed on, but also the good bacteria, called probiotics, that grow during the fermentation process.

Kimchi is a traditional Korean fermented dish often based on cabbage salad. It also contains chilli powder.

Examples of breakfast

Whole grain bread with olive oil, avocado, tomato, cucumber and sprouts.

A bowl of sliced fruit, muesli, nuts, seeds and Proviva (probiotic drink with billions of bacteria). If you prefer a dairy product, choose kefir, which is fermented.

Coffee

water

EXAMPLES OF LUNCH

1-2 whole grain breads with fermented vegetables or kimchi.

Water

EXAMPLES OF DINNER

I'm not a fan of cooking every night, so I make a big meal every Monday that lasts until Thursday.

The food I make contains a lot of healthy vegetables, legumes, soya etc. so I get a natural supply of vitamins, antioxidants, carbohydrates, protein and fat.

I usually vary between a few basic foods and then change the seasoning from week to week. For example, boil red lentils and one week season with curry, cumin and ginger and the next with grated apple, paprika and a little cinnamon. Other spice mixtures are oregano, thyme or rosemary.

In addition to the lentil stew, I usually roast mushrooms, white cabbage, onions, garlic, fennel, root vegetables in the oven and then add to the lentil stew.

· · ·

AN EASY WAY TO get inspiration is to look for recipes for the foods you like and swap meat and fish for good plant-based alternatives. Look at the ingredients to make sure it doesn't contain additives.

You can also search for the dish you're craving and add 'vegan' to the search.

SUMMARY:

Three factors that are already recognized as crucial for our health and that will certainly play an even more important role in the near future are:

1. Microbiota
2. Inflammation in the body.
3. Time-restricted eating (intermittent fasting)

THE DIETARY ADVICE below aims to improve the microbiota and reduce inflammation in the body.

EAT SLOWLY. It takes about 20 minutes for satiety signals to reach the brain. If you eat too fast, you are likely to overeat.

EXERCISE DAILY. You don't have to run a marathon, just walk 7,000-10,000 steps at a brisk pace. It's a good idea to break up your daily walk.

Start by taking daily walks for 15 minutes. Then increase to 30 minutes after 4 weeks. After another 4 weeks, you can increase to 45-60 minutes. After each walk, you should feel that you have done a good job. That feeling alone is enough of a reward.

To AVOID BEING EXPOSED to all the temptations you get when shopping in the supermarket, you can shop online instead. Make a shopping list with only healthy items and stick to it.

32

―――――――――

MEAL SUGGESTIONS

Please accept the repetition from the last chapter, but this is due to the possibility to read each chapter separately.

THESE MEALS SHOULD BE SEEN as suggestions for those who want to change their current diet to one that is a little healthier. If you already eat healthy today, you can of course continue with the diet you eat.

I STARTED CHANGING my diet in the autumn of 2019 and the trigger for me was The game changers on Netflix. Since then, I have gradually modified what I eat according to all the new knowledge I acquire by translating and summarizing scientific studies. What good is knowledge if you don't use it? In my case, it has resulted in these meals, among others.

. . .

As you have read in other chapters, our health is very much about building a good microbiota because it is the engine of our body and controls our health status. Our microbiota needs fibre, so my diet consists largely of fruit, vegetables, root vegetables, legumes, whole grains, nuts and seeds. Of course, you choose what you want to eat, but try to get all these foods into your diet while eliminating ultra-processed foods and drinks.

BREAKFAST

1 sandwich, whole grain sourdough bread.

I bake my own bread to get it the way I want it. It's easy to bake, but I fully understand that it can be difficult to keep up if you are in the middle of life with children, work and various activities.

If you bake buns and cakes, why not swap that baking for baking bread. It's also much healthier.

See the chapter Recipes how to bake bread, make muesli and make a sourdough.

If you buy bread instead, avoid industrial bread, which often contains many additives to improve shelf life, flavor and texture. If you don't want to bake yourself and don't want to buy industrially baked bread, buy bread from a bakery.

TOPPINGS

1-2 tablespoons of olive oil on the bread (contains healthier fat than butter), avocado (a suggestion is frozen to avoid throwing away bad avocado that other customers have damaged by pressing it), cucumber, tomato.

I usually also have sprouts on the sandwich (alfalfa and mung beans are very easy to sprout and minimal risk of failure, will be ready in 4 days).

Bowl of fruit and muesli

I vary the fruit depending on the season and try to avoid fruit from the other side of the world. Apples and unripe bananas both contain good fibre.

I make my own muesli from several different grains. Preferably with the older varieties that have less gluten, but higher protein and fibre content.

Walnuts, hazelnuts, sunflower seeds, pumpkin seeds (depending on price as they can be very expensive).

Instead of milk or plant-based oat or almond drink etc I use a probiotic fruit juice that contains billions of bacteria.

Coffee

Lunch

I don't eat lunch because I am on intermittent fasting or TRE (Time Restricted Eating). Fasting makes me less hungry and my blood sugar is much more stable than before. I also keep the weight off more easily. I use my lunch time to exercise instead.

If you want to eat lunch, bring your own food to work. If you're planning to change your diet, it's a good idea to bring your own food. You can then prepare it when you're not hungry and bring a slightly smaller portion.

Dinner

I, like many others, don't want to cook every night. On Fridays and Saturdays, it's fun to cook together with your loved one.

For that reason, I often choose to make a big batch on Monday that is enough for 4 dinners.

I have no problem eating the same food several days in a row. Because I use many different vegetables, the food is nutritious.

This simple dish is rich in vitamins, fibre, protein, good carbs and good fats.

Red lentils
   Broth
   2 peeled and grated apples. I chop the peel and add it to the soup.

Suggestions for vegetables you can roast in the oven and then add to the soup or stew (depending on how much water you add).

Mushrooms, broccoli, cauliflower, fennel, carrots, parsnips, turnips, celeriac, cabbage or cabbage, onions, leeks, peppers, garlic, lime, sugar, chilli, salt, black pepper.

· · ·

SUGGESTIONS FOR SEASONING

Curry, ground ginger, cinnamon, cumin, cardamom, paprika powder, chilli powder, oregano.

RINSE the lentils first and leave for a while while you prepare the vegetable stew.

CHOP AND SLICE the vegetables and place on baking paper. Drizzle with olive oil, salt and pepper. Put in the oven for 15 minutes at 150 degrees.

BOIL WATER ACCORDING to the instructions for the lentils. Add the broth and a packet of crushed tomatoes. When the water is boiling, add the lentils, grated apples and chopped apple peel. You can also grate the carrot and celeriac and bring to the boil. Cook for just under 8-9 minutes (leave the pot on a low heat). When the soup is ready, add the spices and stir. Finally, add the roasted vegetables.

WEIGHT LOSS PROGRAM – THAT IS SUSTAINABLE

This weight loss program is based on behavioral science studies and research described by The Behavioral Insights Team (BIT), a global organization, started in the UK, that uses behavioral insights to develop models to influence people to make better and wiser decisions (nudging).

IF YOU WANT to change something in your life, such as losing weight or starting to exercise, you are more likely to succeed if you make a plan that you then follow. All change is about building new, sustainable and healthy habits in a structured way. Breaking habitual patterns and behaviors and replacing them with healthier ones.

IN THIS CHAPTER, you will learn how to do this. You will learn why we behave unhealthily and shorten our lives.

How to take command of your brain and teach it good things instead of letting it trick you into making bad decisions. You both direct and play the leading role in your life. And you want it to be an eventful movie with a good and happy ending, right?

In some chapters, the information and message are illustrated with experiments and tests carried out to help you understand the meaning and make it more understandable.

Chapters:

1. DECIDE
2. PLAN
3. COMMITMENT
4. REWARD
5. SHARE
6. FEEDBACK
7. STICK TO

1. DECIDE

Firstly - you need to agree on a few key things to lose weight - you need to be motivated, you need to understand that you really need to lose weight, what losing weight means to you and what you will then be able to do compared to if you don't lose weight.

Lastly and most importantly - you need to keep the weight off over time!

. . .

THIS IS a behavioral science model that will challenge you. A challenge might be that you should lose 12 kg in weight, not 1 kg. That is not a challenge.

BREAK DOWN the end goal into milestones - plan for a gradual weight loss. The more specific the better. If you've decided to lose 12 kg (26 lb) over a year, think of it as losing 1 kg (4,4 lb) per month. This will make the goal much more manageable.

1. Choose the right goal
2. Focus on one goal, set a target and deadline
3. Break down the goal into manageable steps

WRITE a list of what you want/need/must do - like walking 45-60 min per day, eating more fruit and vegetables, not buying sweets, ice cream, soft drinks, energy drinks, changing grocery stores to avoid your habitual routes in the store that always go past the shelves of unhealthy foods, sleeping for 7-8 hours, quitting or reducing alcohol, etc.

Place the list in a strategic place where you are guaranteed to see it, e.g. dining table, toilet. Tick off each item daily as you complete it.

FOR MOST PEOPLE, setting a few goals is rarely a problem. Instead, goals tend to be too many. Few goals give you a better focus.

· · ·

ONCE YOU HAVE DECIDED on a final weight, you need to visualize what your situation might look like and what you will look like when you reach the goal.

Sometimes this can be difficult. When I decided to walk a 800 km (500 miles) pilgrimage route in Spain, it was impossible to realize what it actually means to walk that far distance. We passed a road sign informing 'Santiago de Compostela 790'.

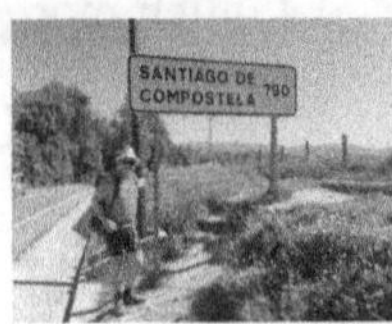

That's right across the north of Spain. In order to complete the walk, I had to break down the daily stages into 30 kilometers (19 miles).

Roncesvalles, Spain
(2015)

WHAT DOES the actual implementation look like in practice? Set a clear goal so you know when you have reached it. Break it down into sub-goals to reach the main goal. Set an end date!

YOUR WEIGHT LOSS efforts start every day as soon as you wake up. A new breakfast. New mindset with more movement. Always try to find opportunities to move and burn calories instead of finding shortcuts to save energy - take the stairs instead of the lift, walk or cycle instead of taking the bus or car. Work out what tasks you need to complete to reach your goal. Be tough but fair to yourself.

. . .

MAKE a shopping list before you go to the supermarket and only buy what is on the list. No spontaneous purchases! If you break this rule, you must pay a large fine (€50 / $50 / £50), which will be donated to a charity organization. Tell someone you know that you will be fined if you break your contract and also when you have been 'fined' so that you do not escape payment.

PLAN when you will exercise and never compromise on time, whatever the weather. Rain and snow are just water. If you are ill, do not exercise! People are lazy by nature so you have to fight it.

PSYCHOLOGISTS HAVE CONCLUDED that it is the interaction between your long-term and short-term goals that is important. The long-term goals help you maintain your drive towards the ultimate goal while the short-term goal creates focus on what you have to do here and now.

THESE THREE RULES will all help you reach your goal:

1. Choose the right goal
Reflect on how your new weight will improve your well-being.

MAKE a list of how your situation is today (example):

1. How much has your weight increased in the last
    few years?
2. Keep a 'diary' for a week and write down
    EVERYTHING you eat and drink, and by
    everything I mean EVERYTHING! If you
    withhold anything, only you will suffer from
    your lie.
3. If you have any health problems?
4. If you have risk factors for disease?
5. If you have a close relative who has fallen ill or
    died prematurely?

THEN GIVE EACH ITEM A 'SCORE' consisting of + and - on a scale of 1-3 based on how good or bad you think you are performing or how bad your health is today. If your weight is very high and you have a high BMI, the score will be -3. If you have no known risk factors (e.g. high cholesterol, high blood pressure), the score will be +3.

The important thing is that you take inventory of your health status and that it becomes clear to you how important it is for you to make a lifestyle change.

IF YOU DO this - and you should spend some time doing it - you will get a good picture of your current situation which should increase your motivation to lose weight and will most likely improve your life.

2. *Focus on a goal, set a target and deadline*
    This point is about making you aware of what your

success looks like, so that once you have reached your goal, it will be clear to you and to those helping you.

3. *Break down the goal into manageable steps*

It is important to break down the main goal into smaller sub-goals. Sub-goals are fundamental. They enable you to see the link between your future main goal and the daily work required of you to get there.

Now THAT YOU have decided on a goal, the chapter Plan will describe how to construct a plan where your daily routines help you make progress towards the goal.

SUMMARY

The three golden rules in this chapter will all help you to achieve your goal. The first rule encourages you to reflect on what is most likely to improve your wellbeing - make a list of the things you want to change in your life and rank them on a scale of 1-10 based on the following two criteria:

1. What effect could it have on your wellbeing

2. How passionate and motivated are you to achieve your goal?

IF YOU DO this - and you should spend some time doing it - you will be well on your way to deciding on a goal that you can take on with passion and that will most likely improve your life.

The second rule is to make yourself aware of what

success looks like, so that it will be clear to you and to those who help you, when you have reached your goal.

Finally, the third rule emphasises the importance of breaking down the main goal into smaller components. These small parts are fundamental to the model. They enable you to see the link between your future main goal and the daily work required of you to get there. Now that you have decided on a goal, the next chapter will describe how to construct a plan where your daily routines help you make progress towards the goal.

2. PLAN

Making a plan is the key factor in helping you reach your goal. And the small details that describe the plan matter a lot. The three rules that will help you get this right are:

1. *Keep it simple* - you should create simple, clear rules that reduce the mental effort required to reach the goal and make you aware of when you are deviating from your goal or the path to get there.

2. *Create an action plan* - you will find that if you outline how, when and where you will carry out the steps, you will increase the chances of success.

3. *Turn the plan into habits* - by repeating the same actions over a period of time, you will create new good habits (and break old ones) making it easier to reach your goal.

1. *Keep it simple*

When you limit your choices, it can be easier to motivate yourself and make decisions.

If you want to lose weight, in addition to simplifying your dietary rules, remove temptations at home and at work.

IF YOU WANT to increase your exercise, try to do it in a simple way, e.g. integrate it with your journey to work (get off a few stops earlier, cycle to work, take the stairs, etc.) or prepare for your workout before you go to bed at night so that it is obvious to you as soon as you wake up or when you get home from work.

Similarly, identify things that may be getting in the way of your goal and remove them.

2. *Create an action plan*

Making it easy and setting clear lines is a first step to creating a simple plan. It will also help you to think about how to proceed to the next step of planning, namely building cognitive links (associations) between moments during the day or week and actions that you have to do.

IMPLEMENTATION INTENTIONS - MEANS intending to change something but failing to carry out the action required to achieve the goal. We are more likely to succeed with our intentions if we can make a cognitive link between the expected future situation and the actions that need to be fulfilled to get there.

For example, if you are going to walk for 45-60 minutes, you should simultaneously decide when to do it, where to go and how long to walk - **WHEN, WHERE, HOW!**

· · ·

To reach a long-term goal, think about how you can trigger the implementation of the activity (special times and places) and do it regularly. When during the day does it fit best (daily routine)?

A trigger could be the alarm clock, toothbrushing or breakfast or when you get home from work - write a list on the breakfast table with prompts such as 'shop for fruit and vegetables', 'get off 1-2 stops before work', 'climb stairs', 'exercise after work' - prepare yourself mentally.

Mental contrasts

Thinking about the benefits of achieving your goals and contrasting them with the obstacles that might get in the way of achieving them.

Example - if I change my eating habits, I will lose weight which will give me better self-confidence and I will dare to show up at the beach next summer.

But you also need to be aware of all the temptations that will come your way, like when you go to a restaurant and choose a healthy dish, it can be easy to fall for a tempting dessert. One tip is to decide in advance to decline the desert menu when the waiter asks and order an espresso or coffee instead. You can even inform the waiter when ordering the main course that you do not want any dessert.

When you combine Implementing Intentions and Mental Contrasts, they become particularly powerful.

Regardless of whether you follow these techniques, the basic premise remains: If you want to achieve your goal, you are more likely to make the change if you first make a plan. And the best way to do that is to create links between elements of your daily routines and actions you need to perform. This will allow you to move from the idea of DOING something (start exercising, eat healthy, lose weight) to the idea of WHEN, WHERE and HOW you are going to do it ('when I get home from work, I'm going to write a shopping list of healthy foods and only buy what's on the list').

If you can create this, you are well on your way to moving from planning to building a habit.

3. Turn the plan into habits

Studies have found that long-term use of various addictive substances was much lower when addicts significantly changed their environment but also that their relapse rate is particularly high when they are exposed to situational reminders related to their previous addiction.

WHEN WE REPEATEDLY EAT SOMETHING RELATED TO a specific environment or situation, our brain will associate that food with that specific situation and make us continue eating as long as we are there. Similarly, if you are going to start shopping for healthy foods, there is a great risk that you will make the usual round in the store and pick up the routine and unhealthy products. One tip might be to change shops. And you should not shop when you are hungry, as this can easily lead to temptation.

. . .

There is a growing consensus that creating habits requires three components:

The first is that habits require a trigger.

The second is that habits require a routine, that the action must be performed (like buying and eating popcorn).

The third and most important is that the routine must be repeated in a consistent context, and it is this repetition that creates an automatic link between the situation you are in and the behavior you perform. This is why habits have the potential to be so powerful, because when behaviors are repeated they do not require active attention or mental effort. Over time, they become automatic reactions, meaning that when we find ourselves in certain situations, we will automatically perform them routinely without conscious control, mental effort or thought.

One of the few studies to investigate the formation of healthy behaviors in real life involved 96 students who were encouraged to repeat behaviors in response to specific reminders (such as taking a walk after breakfast). It was noted that for some students it took 18 days to form a habit while for others it took up to 254 days. For the whole group, it took an average of 66 days.

But what was also noted was that for most, the process of creating a new routine became shorter and shorter until it reached a plateau. In other words, it takes less and less repetition of an action before it becomes a routine.

· · ·

So how can we use habits to achieve our goals? There are three techniques to use depending on whether we want to break old habits, or create new positive ones.

The first is to focus on identifying potential triggers that you use on a daily basis such as the alarm clock, the morning toilet, breakfast, before you leave home, when you arrive at work, etc, and then use these triggers as triggers for your new routines.

What makes this method build a habit is the repetition of the new routine over and over again until a new habit is created.

Repetition in a predetermined context is key - perform the action in the same situation you agreed with yourself to create a habitual behavior (getting off the bus 2 stops earlier, exercising when you get home from work, bringing a lunchbox with new food to work, etc).

The second method is to break reminders that encourage bad habits.

The key to breaking reminders is to think of ways to change your daily environment. If you want to lose weight, get rid of unhealthy foods that you have at home and replace them with foods that help you achieve a more positive eating behavior. An effective strategy to break reminders is to latch onto natural changes in your life. If you change your workplace, take the opportunity to get there in a more exercise-intensive way. Take a broader approach to your change, such as packing a lunchbox with healthy food and traveling to and from work in a more strenuous way.

• • •

THE THIRD WAY involves keeping the reminder steady and not breaking the routine. The first thing to do is to become much more aware of your habitual behavior, which should reduce the propensity to break the habit. In one study, they asked popcorn eaters to eat popcorn with the hand they don't usually use, which resulted in the habitual eaters eating much less popcorn.

The second tactic is to replace a habit with a new one, e.g. snus users use tobacco-free snus instead of nicotine snus.

Note that in these cases, the trigger that sets off the behavior may remain. It is only the response to the trigger that changes. This can be particularly useful in situations where it is difficult to change the response - for example, smoking in stressful situations.

IN MANY WAYS, 'HABITS' are the Holy Grail of behavior change because habits create opportunities for automatic behaviors, and reduce the mental effort required to perform them.

SUMMARY

One of the key lessons learnt is to keep it simple. By setting clear guidelines, you will find that it is easier to stick to your plan and avoid many of the potential setbacks that can occur when introducing new habits.

To help you carry out all the separate actions you need to do, you can use Implementation intentions. This involves thinking about how, when and where you will tackle the tasks you need to complete, which in turn enables you to associate specific mental steps with things you need to do or avoid ('When I get home from work, I'm going to walk for 45 minutes').

AND FINALLY, you can take it to a whole new level by repeating the new actions frequently in those situations where you want to introduce a new healthy behavior. Creating habits makes the task much easier as it reduces the mental effort required to perform an action - especially in the beginning when we see behaviors as chores instead of enjoyable activities.

3. COMMITMENT

Taking on something is relatively easy. But there are a number of things you can do to reinforce the commitment, and increase the likelihood that you will complete it.

THE THREE RULES ARE:

1. Make a commitment - what is it you want to achieve and how are you going to get there - it should be clearly linked to your main goal and to the small sub-goals you will do to get there.

2. Write down the goal and make it public

3. Appoint a 'referee'

1. Make a commitment

A phenomenon most people have experienced is that when they intended to watch an intellectual film, they chose to watch a more light-hearted film instead. An entertaining but quickly forgotten film.

· · ·

IN ONE **EXPERIMENT**, students were divided into 2 groups to watch 3 different films. They wanted to compare whether the participants chose an intellectual or light-hearted film depending on the decision options.

GROUP 1 HAD to choose the film on the day they watched it.

Group 2 had to choose all 3 films on day 1. This meant that on day 1, the conditions between groups 1 and 2 were identical but for days 2 and 3 the choice differed.

THE **RESULTS** SHOWED that most people in group 1 chose light-hearted films each time. Group 2 chose a light-hearted film on day 1, while they chose more intellectual films on the other two occasions.

THIS SIMPLE EXPERIMENT may seem trivial, but it also teaches us something valuable about how we think and reason about the future.

WE TEND to prefer immediate temptations (light-hearted films, hamburgers, chips, computer surfing, video games etc) over 'long-term investments' or benefits (intellectual films, healthy food, getting work documents done, exercising etc), 'because the temptations offer a greater reward in the present'. Behavioral scientists call this 'present bias' - we prefer rewards today to greater gains tomorrow, and therefore postpone difficult decisions and actions, even though we know we shouldn't.

WE PREFER cakes and lying on the sofa today and put off decisions about choosing healthy food and exercising until tomorrow.

We spend today instead of saving for retirement.

We fail to address global issues like climate change because the cost is here and now while the gain is in the future.

IT'S as if we have a present self that prefers ice cream and beer (temptations) and a future self, with different and healthier frames of reference, like abstaining from desserts and preferring to drink water. But the problem is, of course, that at some point our future self will be our current self. And that was exactly the intelligent part of the experiment with the film groups. They showed that it was possible to make our present self think about our future self, and by committing to decisions in advance, it was possible to overcome mental barriers.

THIS IS BASICALLY what a **Commitment Plan** is all about. Your present self makes a promise that binds your future self to make healthier decisions, knowing that in the future it will be your present self that fulfill the promise.

IF YOU REALIZE that you will have trouble making a change (start exercising, eating healthier, lose weight etc) then you should consider making a commitment plan. And such a plan is the important first step.

In the plan, you can link the commitment directly to the main goal (lose 12 kg of weight) and to the demanding actions that need to be done to reach the main goal (exercise 5 times a week, eat more healthy food, avoid sweets, etc). You should also link these commitments to the rewards and punishments you give out depending on your performance.

This is the best way to make your commitments binding and with clear consequences if you fail. If you do all this, you will experience a strong motivation to stick to the promises you made (your contract) and you will feel uncomfortable if you break your commitment. Awareness of the consequences of breaking your promises will help you to stay the course and make the change.

It has been noted that some people who have started shopping for food online do so to avoid temptation and that this way they can shop for food that better suits their future self's preferences. This doesn't include unhealthy food delivery service of course.

2. *Write down your commitment and publish it*
     The first simple step you should do is - write down what it is you are going to do!

· · ·

You can write it down on a piece of paper and put it in front of your designated referee. Writing down your commitment and then signing your promises is an effective way to create consistent behavior. We often do this in the form of employment contracts, marriage papers, purchase documents, etc. These are considered binding and they instruct us to certain commitments, but only when they are created, dated and signed.

Shopping lists also seem to be an effective way to change the way we shop. Not only do they help us remember what to buy, but they also help us avoid impulse purchases, in the same way as shopping for food online - by committing to future actions. So when you've decided to make a change - write it down!

If documenting your change in writing raises the stakes, publishing will turbocharge it. In other words, you should not keep your commitment to yourself.

Writing down a commitment in advance and making it public creates a stronger incentive to implement the change than if we just think about implementing it.

Writing down the change we plan to make creates social pressure on us to live up to our own expectations about our behavior. When we publish our commitment it means exposing our internal pressure to others. It is how sustainable our character is in the eyes of others that is important to us.

If, in addition to publicizing your commitment, you add how you will go about achieving it (publicly), you increase your chances of success. This is the hallmark of a Commitment Plan.

In this strategy, it is important to link your commitment to your plan and to your goal.

3. *APPOINT A 'REFEREE' to your commitment*

An example comes from a comedy show where one person asks another person to be her 'dessert referee' and stop her from eating dessert no matter what!

THE PERSON REALIZED two things - firstly, that her future self would be at risk of falling for temptation and secondly, that in order to accomplish the task, she had to appoint a referee who would stop her NO MATTER WHAT!

IF YOU WANT to achieve your goal, you have to realize the importance of appointing a referee who will follow your change process and who is not afraid to make unpopular decisions if you fail in your mission and to impose a predetermined penalty (see https://stickk.com which is a US service focused on Commitment). Data from Stickk.com shows that appointing a referee increases the likelihood of successful change. If you do, you are 70% more likely to succeed with your change compared to those who do not appoint a referee.

THERE ARE two factors that are important when choosing a referee:

1. That the referee is fair and does not conspire against the person to make them fall for a temptation.
2. That the referee has the courage to stand up and is not afraid to hand out both punishment and reward if the commitment is followed or not followed. The person you are in a relationship with is probably not perfect as a referee, as being harsh can put a strain on the relationship.

THEREFORE, avoid both an enemy and a good-hearted friend as a referee.

- Write an agreement
- Make it public / publicized
- Appoint a referee who is tough but fair

SUMMARY

Instruments of engagement are useful because our present self seems to have different preferences than our future self. If we were not aware of this conflict, it would be difficult to engage in anything. But thankfully, humans seem to be fully aware of their weaknesses, which is why so many people lock themselves into options that bind future actions - like opening savings accounts that remain closed until we reach our savings goal.

These instruments work, first of all, because we are prepared to enter into them because we are aware of our problem of lack of self-control. Once we have made a commitment, we put pressure on ourselves to be consistent with the promise we have made, knowing that it strengthens our commitment.

By writing down our commitment and publicizing it, we not only increase the pressure on ourselves to be consistent with the promise, we also feel external pressure to do so. And this can be further increased if you appoint a referee - someone who supports you and doesn't pull you down - but who can stand up and impose punishment when you break the pledge or don't fulfill what you promised. The referee is also the one who can decide whether the reward should be paid or not.

4. REWARD

All economic textbooks show that changes in the costs or benefits of doing something will change behavior.

Rewards help activate specific pathways in our brain, which not only make us feel good, but also encourage us to look for further rewards.

But what works in some situations does not work at all in others.

THREE INGREDIENTS for designing reward systems that encourage people to reach their goals are:

1. Put something valuable at stake
2. Use small rewards to build good habits
3. Watch out for setbacks

GOLD STARS and smileys work as rewards for young children but are rather ineffective for older children.

A FINANCIAL REWARD needs to be targeted at the right goal to have the desired effect and offered in a context where it increases motivation.

1. Put something meaningful at stake - bet on something
Link a significant reward to reaching your goal, make it binding and enforce it.

SMOKERS in the Philippines (Project CARES) who wanted to quit smoking set aside the same amount they spent on cigarettes for 6 months. The money was deposited in a bank account. The people were continuously tested with a urine dipstick to see if they smoked and if so, the money saved went to charity.

The results after 6 months showed that those in the program quit smoking at a higher rate - 30% - than the control group. At the 12-month follow-up, there were also more non-smokers in the active group than in the control group.

THERE ARE 4 simple tips to help create an effective reward system.

1. There needs to be a clear line between the reward you set aside and your ultimate goal.

In other words - your reward is only paid out if you reach your goal! The easiest way is to link the reward to your commitment. In your commitment, you should describe what your goal is and when you will have reached it (date).

IF YOU WANT to lose 12 kg (26 lb), make it clear that the reward will only be paid if you reach the target weight and if you do so by the deadline.

No reward will be paid if you almost reach the weight, nor will you get 'another week' to do it.

2. It must be a meaningful reward - 'Pay enough or not at all' - Professor Dean Karlan, Behavioral Economist, Yale University.

THE STAKES MUST BE high enough to have the desired effect. Dean Karlan and a friend challenged each other to lose weight. The stakes were half a year's salary. The reason for the high sum was that every time he went to the freezer for ice cream he would be aware of what he was jeopardizing. They both managed to reach their target weight.

It doesn't have to be half a year's salary as a reward, nor does it have to be a financial reward.

But if the price you pay for reaching your goal is not valuable enough, it will not motivate you to try to make the change.

In addition, Karlan has set $5000 at stake to ensure that he maintain his new weight. In 6 years, he has not lost any money. And his life expectancy has increased by almost five years.

3. The reward must be binding

You must realize that the reward will only be paid if you manage to implement the change. If you try to change or rewrite the initial contract, you are considered to have failed.

In short - there should be no way out of the contract.

The best way to enforce your binding contract is to appoint a referee to help you through the change process.

4. Construct the contract according to the loss aversion principle, i.e. it should hurt to lose

According to repeated experiments, it has been found that the feeling of losing is twice as strong as the feeling of winning. For example, we feel worse when we lose €100 than we feel good when we find the same amount.

2. Use small rewards to create good habits.

Motivate yourself during the change process by using small incentives linked to specific steps necessary to reach the end goal.

. . .

EXPERIMENT:

Timboon, a town in Australia, recognised that its residents were becoming overweight and inactive. The local health authority along with a team of behavioral scientists were well aware that small rewards can be powerful in creating good daily habits. They conducted the test on the health authority staff. Everyone was given a Fitbit watch (fitness watch) and tasked with walking 10,000 steps per day.

AFTER A WHILE, it was noticed that the number of steps started to decrease.

They then divided the people into groups and offered each of them a voucher worth €50 if everyone in the group increased the number of steps by 2,500 steps per day.

RESULT: The number of steps per week increased by 2,100 in average. It was also noted that those who needed it most increased the most in both steps and calories burned.

It helps to break down your final goal into smaller sub-goals. Then link smaller rewards to the sub-goals. These types of sub-goals will help you reach your main goal.

EXAMPLE: If you want your child to clean their room, start by rewarding them for picking up ONE toy. Then 5 toys, etc. The rewards should be of the 'Good job' type and help to create good habits and behaviors when linked to daily routines.

· · ·

EXPERIMENT:

In several elementary schools in the United States, they wanted to get children to eat more fruit and vegetables. All children who took fruit and vegetables were given a ticket worth $2.50. These could only be redeemed in the school shop, during the school carnival or in the bookshop. Not for sweets, cakes or similar. One group was followed up for 3 weeks and another group for 5 weeks. They were interested in seeing what happened AFTER the test, i.e. whether the behavior was permanent and had become a habit.

RESULTS: 2 months after the end of the test, both groups had increased their intake of fruit and vegetables, but the effect in the 5-week group was twice as large, i.e. they ate twice as much fruit and vegetables as the 3-week group. Repetition of a behavior creates habits. The longer the period of repetition, the stronger the behavior becomes and the easier it becomes a habit.

Linking a competitive element to the goal, by rewarding milestones but also by exposing them to competition, increases the power of implementation.

WHEN THE AMERICAN vegetable test was repeated in England, stickers worth £2.50 were used instead. The children could save 4 and redeem them for a toy and this method achieved the same results.

But when they added a competitive element by dividing the children into groups of 4 and only those with the most stickers received a reward - fruit and vegetable intake increased by 3 times!

. . .

In addition to main goals, sub-goals and rewards, adding a competitive element (against yourself or others) ultimately helps to create new, better and healthier habits.

It's not really losing weight, or stopping smoking, or starting to exercise that is the end goal - IT'S CREATING THE HABIT THAT MAKES YOU CONTINUE WITH THE NEW BEHAVIOR!

3. Watch out for setbacks

Financial incentives can knock out the intrinsic motivation that is already there. So be aware that rewards and punishments can undermine good intentions. Instead, you can use different types of non-financial rewards.

Don't try to reward good social deeds. If you are initially motivated to perform an action, a financial reward is not always perceived as something positive.

Experiment:

Collecting money for charity.

Group 1 was told that the people who raised the most money would be presented in public.

Group 2 was told the same but with the addition that they would receive 1% of the money raised.

Group 3 was told the same but that they would receive 10% of the money raised.

· · ·

RESULTS:

Group 1 was the most successful (without financial incentive) and shortly after came Group 3 (10% of money raised).

Last and 36% worse, came Group 2 who were offered the low commission (1%).

RAISING money for charity has an inherent power that is highly motivating. Trying to replace it with an external force in the form of a low commission led to a much lower motivation to perform a good deed.

ANOTHER STUDY STARTED FINING parents who were late picking up their children from daycare. With the result that the parents paid up!

THEN THEY TRIED REMOVING the fine and the result was that the parents continued to pick up late. They had created the behavior that it is okay to 'sell' their morals. The parents had created immoral behavior.

IF YOU WANT to use a financial incentive - make it attractive and meaningful!

ON THE OTHER HAND, if you set the price too high, it risks not being cost-effective, or worse, it encourages cheating, dishonesty or poor performance. The target must be achievable, otherwise you risk having no effect at all - people won't care.

INSTEAD OF PROVIDING financial rewards where there is intrinsic motivation, there are three other approaches.

THE FIRST APPROACH says that it is not always best to give cash rewards. Instead, it may be wise to focus on what the sum can offer you - a trip, a product, an event, a dinner, a holiday, etc.

IN A STUDY from Singapore to get taxi drivers to train more, taxi drivers were given a choice between an offer of $1,000 or paying for a day's rental of their taxi.

THE OFFER TO pay for a day was by far more effective. Surprising? The lease cost for one day was also $1,000. This shows that in some cases you should focus on what the money can give you or the person you are offering the reward.

IT IS ALSO SHOWN that those who receive money donated in their name instead of cash for themselves, were more satisfied and happy.

THE SECOND METHOD is related to the first and is particularly suitable when offering rewards to others. It departs from the principle of cash rewards and instead offers services, events, that they would never otherwise receive.

EXAMPLE: Electric cars in Oslo are allowed to drive in the lane for buses and taxis, which has had a huge impact on the number of electric cars sold. Today, there are so many electric cars in Oslo that this benefit has been cancelled, which shows the power of the offer.

ANOTHER EXAMPLE IS HANDING out pens labelled with names and years, as an annual reward. Cheap and desirable.

THE THIRD METHOD can be called anti-incentive - you set aside money as a reward for successful change and achievement of goals, but if you fail, it is paid to another person, organisation, political party, etc. that you dislike.

In the case of financial bets and anti-incentives, the amount does not need to be very large - losing money to someone or something you dislike is particularly painful.

BUT BE aware that the agreement should be binding - no backing out - which means you MUST implement the change you promised.

SUMMARY

To achieve your goal, ensure that ALL overall rewards are meaningful by focusing on 4 key principles:

1. There is a direct link between the reward and the overall goal.
2. The reward must be meaningful enough that you really care about achieving the goal.
3. Make sure the reward is tied to the goal.
4. Design the contract so that you lose something when you don't reach the goal (instead of gaining something) - the discomfort of losing something (loss aversion) is a stronger incentive than the pleasure of gaining something (losing a larger amount of money compared to finding the equivalent amount).

Be aware that financial rewards can undermine an already existing and intrinsic motivation. Ways to minimize this risk are to design the incentives in the contract carefully, rewarding you with experiences rather than money, or to create an anti-incentive contract - if you fail, the money set aside goes to someone or something you dislike or you have to do something you perceive as humiliating, such as walking down the main street wearing only underwear. If your goal is to lose 12 kg in a year, with milestones of 1 kg per month, and if at each monthly weigh-in you fail to lose 1 kg, you are fined a certain amount of money for something you don't like.

Also consider group incentives - helping each other, pressurizing everyone in your group to contribute to your goal or competing against other groups will increase the chances of you working harder and reaching your goal.

. . .

5. SHARE

Behaviors are contagious. For example, if you want to quit smoking - socialize with non-smokers. If you want to lose weight, socialize with people who encourage you, not people who want to drag you into doing something unhealthy.

SITUATIONS, surroundings, places, friends etc trigger behaviors. Avoid places or situations that trigger your cravings for bad things when making a change - going to a pub and drinking beer may not be the best place to quit smoking. Not only does it impair your judgement, but beer and alcohol also trigger your cravings.

IT IS SAID that a problem shared is a problem halved, and the same can be said for achieving goals - they are often easier to achieve if we share them with others - in different ways.

PUBLICISE YOUR GOAL, use groups, bring your partner, friend, colleague to help you lose weight, ask friends for help, social contacts, etc.

- Ask for help
- Share in your social network
- Use group power (alone is not strongest)

EXAMPLE: If a spouse quits smoking, it has been shown that in 67% of cases the partner also quits.

GET help from others to reach your goal. If you share that you are going to make a change, others can provide motivation and support you in the process.

IF YOU ASK someone for a favour, it triggers a strong urge in you to reciprocate. Darwin recognised that one of the pillars of morality is 'the power of repayment'.

WE ARE SOCIAL ANIMALS. We are influenced by what other people do and what they think of us. Often unconsciously and to a much higher degree than we are aware of.

THE 3 RULES TO use to get the most out of the social components are:

1. Ask for help; this increases the chances of you reaching your goal.
2. Engage your social contacts; powerful effect on our behaviors.
3. Use the power of group interaction; if more people strive to reach the same goal, the chances of success increase compared to doing it on your own.

1. Ask for help

In repeated experiments, it has been found that 50% of people surveyed were willing to help total strangers.

Imagine then how many friends and acquaintances are willing to help us.

EXAMPLE:

When parents received text messages from the teacher with specific information about upcoming homework and exams, it resulted in better co-operation between parents and children. It also resulted in an improved study result equivalent to 1 month of study.

ANOTHER VERY EFFECTIVE learning method is to let pupils tutor each other, good pupils help those who are struggling. It has also been found that we learn better from those similar to ourselves (e.g. children learn to swim faster by watching other children, compared to learning from a swimming teacher - 'if they can do it, so can I').

HEALTH PROGRAMMES TO STOP SMOKING, drink less, lose weight, start exercising, which offer group programmes work better than individual programmes.

IF WE EXERCISE with someone else instead of exercising alone, we exert ourselves more, get more exercise, exercise for longer time, etc. The competitive element increases our commitment. Find a person and think about how to ask them for help - what kind of help and when.

. . .

2. Engage your social contacts

In 1940, Lego started producing its products in plastic. Things gradually improved and from 1978 the company doubled in size every five years. In 2004, things started to go downhill fast as toy companies found it difficult to compete with digital products. But Lego managed to turn the tide, thanks in large part to the amazing network of Lego users it had built up over the years.

In 2008, they started 'Lego ideas', which meant that users could submit proposals for new products. You upload your proposal to a website. After that, Lego needs 10,000 people to support your suggestion over a two-year period for Lego to develop 'your' product. At the same time, Lego has received confirmation (market research) that the market will buy the product. When Minecraft supporters launched the idea of a Lego based on the computer game, it took 2 days to get 10,000 supporters - Lego Minecraft Micro was in stores 6 months later.

Another example is the Apple Support Community where users help each other with problems without Apple getting involved.

When it comes to obesity, rates vary widely between countries. Obesity travels through social networks. The risk of becoming overweight is 45% higher if the people around you are overweight compared to if they are of normal weight.

. . .

3. Use and harness the power of groups

More and more individuals are quitting smoking and the number of 'smoking groups' (the collective pattern of smoking in groups during breaks) is also decreasing. However, the size (number of people in the group) of smoking groups remains almost constant. This means that people quit smoking in groups - when one or more people in the group decide to quit, more people join in.

EXAMPLE:

The Weight Watchers program compared group weight loss with individual implementation.

RESULTS: Members who lost weight in a group lost an average of 5 kg (11 lb) and those who completed an individual program lost 2.25 kg (5 lb).

EXAMPLE:

Saving money - group savings, where the amount saved was then presented publicly, were compared with individual savings, where people also received a higher interest rate (5% individual savings compared to 0.3% in group savings).

RESULT: Group savers doubled their savings and the higher interest rate hardly affected the savings of individual savers at all.

· · ·

It is said that a problem shared is a problem halved, and the same can be said for reaching our goals - they are often easier to reach if we share them with others, by using groups, asking friends for help, social contacts, etc.

SUMMARY

Behaviors are contagious.

If you want to lose weight, you should surround yourself with people who are not overweight. Studies have shown that if you socialise with people who are overweight, you are more likely to become overweight yourself than if you socialise with people of normal weight.

It is also important to surround yourself with people who encourage you, and not people who want to drag you into unhealthy behavior.

Situations, surroundings, places, friends etc trigger behaviors. Avoid places or situations that trigger your cravings when making a change - going to a pub for a pint may not be the best place to stop smoking or lose weight. Not only does it impair your judgement, but beer triggers cravings for salty peanuts and crisps. And smoking.

They say that a problem shared is a problem halved. It is often easier to achieve a set goal if you implement a change together with others. And there is double the joy when everyone is on target.

Publicise your goals, get help from groups, bring your partner, friend or colleague along when you want to lose weight, ask friends for help, social contacts, etc.

. . .

6. FEEDBACK
Experiment:

In England, it was noted that the prescription of antibiotics increased significantly. As a result, the risk of resistant bacterial strains increased.

In an attempt to influence GPs to reduce their prescribing, the following was done: information on prescribing in health centers was collected and doctors in the top 20% of prescribers were identified.

Half of the doctors received a letter telling their prescribing patterns and 3 concrete tips on how they could change their prescribing - a delayed prescription i.e. the patient can collect the medicine if symptoms persist; how their prescribing compared to other doctors; information that 80% of GPs in their area prescribe less antibiotics than they do.

The other half received no letter or information.

RESULTS: After six months, the doctors who received the letter and advice had prescribed 73,400 FEWER prescriptions than those who did not receive a letter.

THERE WAS no change in the strength of the antibiotic. No financial incentives for doctors. No mass mailings from the centre lecturing them. Just pure feedback and tips on what they could do.

. . .

It's hard to know how close you are to your goal if you don't know how you are performing and where you are right now. Good feedback is not only about knowing where you stand, it is also about knowing what you can do to perform better, and recognizing what is possible to do by knowing how others are performing compared to how you are performing.

Unfortunately, we often fail to gather information and provide continuous feedback.

The 3 rules for feedback are:

1. Find out where you are in relation to where you are going - your goal.
2. Feedback continuously and at set times, feedback with specific information, itemised, personalized and focused on the effort required (ideally you want personalized feedback, knowing what you need to do to reach the goal and it should be linked in time to the achievement).
3. Compare your performance with others - if possible, find out how well you perform in comparison with others. In some situations this can be the most powerful feedback of all!

1. Find out where you are in relation to where you are going - your goal.

Play the game '*Hot or cold*'. The important principle of

good feedback is to know where things are in relation to where you should be.

EXAMPLE: Each additional star (based on guest ratings - feedback) for a restaurant on the consumer search service Yelp increased profits in the following year by 5-9%.

EXAMPLE: Students training were divided into three groups.

Group 1 set a goal to increase their performance by 40% compared to their last training session, but they received no feedback on their performance.

Group 2 received feedback on how they performed compared to their last session, but they did not set a goal on how they wanted to perform.

Group 3 set goals and received continuous feedback.

RESULT: Group 3 doubled their performance compared to the other two groups.

In other words, information alone is not enough.

WE ARE OFTEN PRESENTED with goals to achieve. But we rarely have the opportunity to step back and reflect on the progress we are making towards the goal, what is successful and what is not.

When considering your goals, look for information that allows you to know where you are in relation to where you are going.

· · ·

If **you want to lose weight** - decide your ultimate target weight and decide what you need to do and what efforts are required to get there (diet, exercise, temptations, traps, realisation of hard work etc).

Feedback not only shows us what we are doing wrong, it also allows us to better understand the impact and success we are making in relation to our main goal. We humans like to feel that we are making progress, so we should think about designing feedback systems that maximize that feeling.

Experiment: A café compared two variants of loyalty cards. One with 10 squares to be stamped to get a free cup of coffee. The other with 12 squares, but with the first two already stamped with 'Bonus'. 10 squares still had to be stamped. Both variants of cards thus involved the same number of purchases to get a free cup of coffee.

Results: The card pre-stamped with 'Bonus' led to significantly better results. The reason was that people perceived that they had already made progress towards the goal. And once you have started, you want to continue. The risk is otherwise that you are filled with the feeling that you have spent money on something 'unnecessarily'.

2. Provide feedback continuously and at set times
    Example: Roadside displays showing current speed have been shown to reduce speed 10% better than other

models such as 'slow down' signs, fines or speed cameras etc. The reasons are: you get immediate feedback on your speed compared to a fine two months later; you get personalized feedback; it is correctable (you can reduce speed immediately).

EXPERIMENT: The theory that children who are told they have an innate talent for maths, for example, are likely to be devastated if they fail, with the consequence that they will not want to take on challenging tasks.

CHILDREN WERE DIVIDED into 2 groups. First, they had to do a task where they were told that they had performed well (at least 80% correct).

One group received feedback that the reason they did so well was because they were smart.

The other group was told that the reason they had done so well was because they had worked hard.

In the next task, everyone was told that they had performed poorly (no more than 50% correct). Then they wanted to see how the children reacted to the negative criticism with a third task.

Although the 'smart' children were familiar with the tasks they were doing, they performed much worse, while those who had been encouraged to work hard improved significantly.

HARD WORK PAYS OFF!

THERE ARE two types of attitude - an 'ingrained attitude' and a 'developing attitude'.

'Ingrained attitude' - we believe that our qualities are set in stone, which results in us constantly having to assert ourselves.

'Developing attitude' - we believe that our basic qualities can be developed through our efforts.

Instead of praising people for having inherent qualities or talent, effort and persistence in solving tasks should be encouraged.

3. Compare your performance to others

We care a lot about how others perceive us. We compare ourselves to others and we are strongly influenced by what those around us do and say. This is called the social norm - the values, actions and expectations of a specific social group, and it offers a guide to our behavior.

MAKING people aware of what the majority does is called Descriptive Social Norm - it can reinforce an underlying motivation. And there is a good reason for that. Not only are we humans strongly influenced by the behavior of others, we are also often unaware of what other people are really doing, and we are prone to undervalue the good behaviors of others. Instead, we think they cheat on their taxes, eat unhealthily and don't exercise much.

And this creates an opportunity - by understanding and communicating what the prevailing social norm is or what they do, we can motivate ourselves and others.

EXAMPLE: To get more people to pay their taxes in England, three different messages were used:

'Nine out of ten pay their tax on time' - was effective.

'The vast majority of people in your area pay their taxes on time' - was even more effective.

'The majority of people with a similar tax debt to yours have already paid their taxes' - was most effective!

EXPERIMENT: Step competition in Australia. People were divided into 50 groups.

The groups were given two different messages.

Half of the groups were told which group had walked the most steps.

The other half were told how their own group performed, i.e. what place they were in, how far away (number of steps) they were from the leader group and who was most efficient in their group.

The groups that received detailed information performed better and, most importantly, those who had walked the least number of steps in the groups improved.

ALL PEOPLE CARE about how they perform compared to others (and especially compared to their peers). Athletes don't just care about their times, they care about how they perform compared to others.

ONE STUDY FOUND that Olympic silver medallists were less satisfied than bronze medallists because they were so close to winning gold.

The bronze medallists were satisfied because they had made the podium at all and avoided the humiliating fourth place.

. . .

THE SAME IS true in professional life - we care less about what our salary is. Instead, we care more about whether it is higher or lower than that of our colleagues doing the same job.

WHEN WE HAVE to achieve a difficult goal, we not only want to know how well we are doing, we also care about and are motivated by whether others are performing better or worse than we are.

SUMMARY

Today, there are a lot of tools - apps and other digital tools - that give you feedback on how you are performing.

But this information alone won't help you much - you need to know where you are in relation to where you are going, i.e. your goal. You also need to be aware of what you can do to perform even better next time.

For these reasons, feedback at set times, which is specific, personalized and focuses on effort (rather than innate talent) is very useful. It helps you understand what you can do with the information you receive. We also know that if you can compare YOUR performance with the performance of OTHERS, you will probably reach your goal faster.

7. STICK TO

If you want to reach a future goal, you need to be

prepared to work hard; to put in effort and practice; and to learn from both successes and failures along the way.

WHEN SETTING a personal goal for the distant future, you need to start by setting sub-goals to be achieved first - TO ACHIEVE ANYTHING BIG, YOU MUST FIRST WIN THE SMALL SUB-GOALS!

THIS CHAPTER IS about how to use the techniques in the previous chapters to stay focussed towards our future goal (and not to go astray).

3 RULES TO stick to in order to reach a goal are:

1. Practice with focus and effort - if you need to improve your performance over time to reach your goal, be aware that the quality of the training is as important as the quantity i.e. the time you spend on it.
2. Learn by testing - once you have broken down your goals into smaller and achievable steps, you can improve your performance by testing what works best - test and evaluate small changes (what works and what doesn't).
3. Reflect and celebrate success - when you find out what works and what doesn't, don't forget to celebrate your achievements before moving on.

1. Practice with focus and effort

We all have the ability to improve in different areas, but if you want to be at the top of your game in one area - sport, music etc - you need to put in >10,000 hours, but those hours MUST include quality.

If you want to lose weight, both your elaborate plan and your work to reach first the intermediate goals and then your final weight will be your training to maintain the weight over time. If you are careful with the preparation, the execution will go better.

2. Learn by testing

Break down your goal into sub-goals. Test yourself and see what works by starting with the question 'Does it work?' every time you try something new.

EXAMPLE: If I write a letter to people telling them how many have already paid their taxes, does it work? YES.

IF I SEND a message to people with a picture of their house lit up in infrared color showing how much energy they use and compare it to a picture of the house without infrared color, will it get more people to insulate their homes? NO. It will instead reduce the number of households that insulate their homes, as most people think that red shimmering houses look cosy.

GOOGLE TESTED and found that just a small change to the

blue color in the toolbar increased advertising revenue by $20 billion.

THE THREE HARDEST words to say might be 'I don't know'. In almost all areas (work, leisure, exercise etc.) we are failing by not knowing what works and what doesn't. Unfortunately, large sums are invested in expensive projects where you don't know if it works or not because you don't test and evaluate.

IN ORDER TO change and test what really works, you need to be aware and admit to yourself that you do not know best, that you are not the best at implementing, that you do not behave in the best way etc and that you are willing to make a change. You need to be positive about trying different options to see what works best for you.

EXAMPLE: If you want to burn more calories, compare walking to work with going by bus to work. Take the stairs 4 floors compared to riding the lift. And then do both (walking to work + taking the stairs) and see what burns the most calories.

There are mobile apps and fitness apps that measure calorie burning. For example, the Health app, available for both iPhone and Android. Set your personalized parameters such as weight and height and it will give you reliable feedback.

3. Reflect and celebrate success

Reflect on what you have achieved in reaching your goal - have you had any (positive) impact on other people's lives? Has your work to change your weight rubbed off on a friend or colleague?

IF YOU LOST weight and started exercising, reflect on what you learnt along the way.

EXPERIMENT: In a call centre in India, all new employees received the same technical training, but with one crucial difference: one group set aside 15 minutes at the end of each working day to reflect and write down their experiences of the day's work.

The other group worked on as usual. In the final test, those who reflected daily performed on average 20% better than those who had not.

As YOU WORK on your weight loss, at the end of your day, reflect on how you think your change is affecting you positively and negatively. Can you change the things you perceived as negative?

By reflecting, you can mentally prepare for tomorrow and what you will then work on. Feel free to write down how you envision that work.

When you wake up the next morning, briefly review what you wrote down the night before. You are preparing to win the battle against your interim goal every day.

. . .

You should continuously reflect on the path towards your goal when you make progress, but also when you have setbacks. Think about what you have learnt along the way - use this information when deciding how to proceed, what to try next (daily personal feedback).

Reflect also when you reach the final destination. Also plan how you want to celebrate when you reach your final goal.

There is a psychological reason to do so, especially if the path to the goal has been demanding. It relates to a little-known psychological construct called the 'Peak-End rule' - where people judge an experience based on how they felt at the end of the experience, and when the feeling was at its most intense, rather than the total sum of the pleasure or pain the experience gave us.

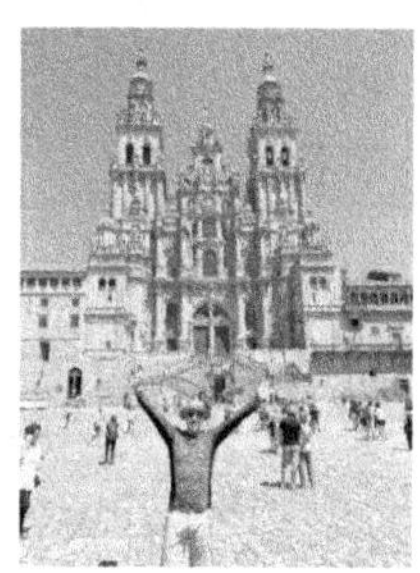

Finish line after the Camino Primitivo (325 km or 202 miles) at the Cathedral of Santiago de Compostela, Spain

Experience and memory are different things and our evaluation of experience is dominated by the pleasure or discomfort we experience most at the end of the event.

This means that we should think about how to mitigate moments of discomfort and maximize the peaks of pleasure and enjoyment, and ensure that the final moments when we are about to reach our goal are as pleasurable and enjoyable as possible. Celebrate these moments - a dinner, a hotel weekend, traveling etc.

It helps you remember why you went through a year of hard work to reach your goal. It helps you focus on the positive part of the work and not on the difficult, stressful and negative part, and it makes you more willing to take on new challenges.

During the 2020 pandemic, I bought a bike to combine vacation and exercise. The plan was to cycle to my sister and brother-in-law, a journey of 270 km. The route I drew up in maps I bought, but also in Google maps which is actually better than in paper maps. At least as long as your mobile phone is connected. What I discovered already after a few hours on the bike was that, based on the map, I did not realize how hilly and demanding the road was.

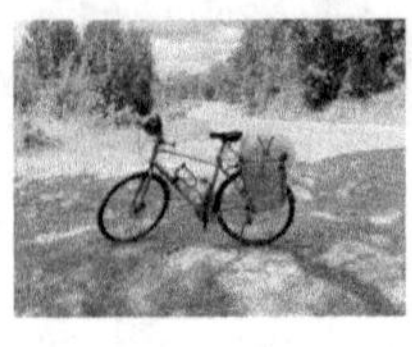

Energy break during 1st day of my hilly tour 2020.

You don't recover from a steep uphill by rolling down a long downhill. At least not if the journey goes up and down for several hours. And with 2 heavy panniers on the rack.

After these 2 days of demanding cycling, I needed 5 days for recovery before I could continue the final 540 km.

The last part was not nearly as physically demanding as the first 270 km were.

I remember expressing loud and clear that I would never cycle that distance again. Now that a few years have passed, I realize that my brain seems to have repressed how demanding it was and secretly (without my active participation) started planning to cycle the same distance again. And I have to actively resist so as not to start planning another bike ride that route.

SUMMARY

When we set out to achieve a goal, and especially a future goal that requires us to learn new skills over time, it's easy to just rush off and repeat behaviors we've always done.

If we do this, we will find that we are not actually learning. For example, we might think we are exercising if we walk slowly for 20 minutes while talking on the phone. Or adding a bowl of green salad with vinaigrette to your meal without removing unhealthy elements from your diet. Then we are not exercising and we are not eating healthy, but we only experience the feeling that we are doing so.

But if we really want to get better at a task over time, we need to think about how to TEACH ourselves to do it. And the best way to do that is to first figure out how we're going to make the change - by breaking down our goals and focusing on making incremental improvements in how we do the task.

· · ·

THIS METHODOLOGY WILL MAKE you realize that testing and experimenting with new ideas and technologies comes to you more naturally. You will learn from the feedback you receive along the way, and by testing small changes - one at a time - to see what effect they have on your weight loss.

Finally, once you start to achieve success, even if you encounter some setbacks along the way, you need to take time to reflect on what seems to be working for you and what isn't (what is stopping you from making progress). When losing weight, you will find that you lose relatively many kilos quickly, but that the weight loss can suddenly stop. Evolution has designed our bodies not to burn calories, but to save energy for days when food may be scarce. You can then try new diet and exercise options and see if they help you lose weight again.

CONCLUSION

If you have a goal that is some way off in the future, the chances of reaching it are reduced if you don't break it down into milestones. To reach a big goal, you must first create and overcome the small goals.

THE SCIENCE **behind**

To understand why thinking small makes sense, we need to understand the science behind how we make decisions - the importance of understanding how we humans process information and make decisions.

OUR BRAIN HAS A SLOW, reflective system and a fast, automatic system.

The slow system helps us when we learn new things, like when we learn to drive a car. The fast system then allows us to drive the car with ease, handle all the instruments and navigate from A to B.

THE KEY to making this model of change work, with its main goal and several smaller sub-goals, is to understand how and when to switch on the slow system, and how and when to encourage the fast system to take over. This is not easy, because although the fast system makes our lives easier in a complex world (all our habitual behaviors like driving, traveling to work, doing daily chores like housework, taking care of our hygiene, etc.), the automatic system is also prone to systematic errors.

AT THE SAME TIME, our brain does not have enough mental power to let the reflective system make all the decisions. We have a limited mental bandwidth and we will fail if we ask for more than our concentration can handle. This is why the small details are so important.

CREATING small sub-goals helps us to achieve our big goals by utilizing the strengths of both the fast and slow systems and avoiding the pitfalls of each.

ONE OF THE most important descriptions of how the two systems work in practice is to understand their effect of 'time'.

The fast system has a strong preference for immediate

(here and now) rewards and prefers to postpone difficult and thoughtful decisions until later.

Our slow system understands that there may be more appropriate and correct choices to make, but only if the reward is delayed until later ('tomorrow') and that other and more challenging decisions need to be addressed today.

Several of the tools in the methodology of this change model focus on getting us to make more morally correct decisions and to see the fast-paced system as a resource and friend and not as an enemy.

CREATE small goals and reach far

You don't have to use all 7 parts in every situation, but the more you use, the stronger the 'scaffolding' becomes. Just like any other structure, you start by laying the foundation. It starts with HOW you decide on your goal. Then, at a deeper level, engage your reflective system. Spend time thinking about the goal you primarily want to achieve. What does it mean for you to lose weight? What will you be able to do then that you cannot do today? What health benefits will you get when you lose weight?

BREAKING your goal down into more manageable steps will help you reach it faster. Then plan how you will reach your goal. Use an 'if-then plan', which means you link deliberate actions to specific steps in your daily routine.

BY REPEATING these new actions every time you get the 'signal' (like Pavlov's dogs), you can start to develop habits to automate actions that were previously exhausting and challenging. Slowly but surely, you'll notice your fast system taking over more and more.

Then you use the tools you have been given (to further strengthen your 'scaffolding') to keep yourself motivated.

In the chapter on **Commitment**, you learnt how to overcome the tension we all feel about our present and future selves. By writing down your goal and publicizing it, it makes you more motivated to get all the way to your end goal - we compete against our shame of failure.

Reward systems can be very effective, but they can also backfire if you don't get the small details right.

Striving to reach a goal seems to many to be a purely individual improvement project. But working with others not only makes the work more enjoyable, it also increases the chances of success.

Feedback is crucial - it's very difficult to achieve something if you don't know how you're performing along the way. You need to be continuously informed about where you are on the path to your goal. For example, if you want to lose 12 kg and you have an intermediate goal of losing 1 kg every month, you need to check your weight every month. If you check your weight only after 6 months and it turns out that you have only lost 3 kg, you have deviated from your plan.

To further strengthen the 'scaffolding', we need to put a lot of effort into training and honing our skills, testing and experimenting to find out what works best to reach our end goal but also to find out what doesn't work.

And finally, take time to reflect and celebrate when you reach your goal. Not only to reap the rewards of your hard work but also to learn for future tasks.

"Skill breeds skill ' - Professor James Heckman.

In other words, when you have successfully achieved your goal, you have learnt how to construct a 'scaffolding' to reach future goals. This is useful when you set a new goal. Or if you are helping others to make a lifestyle change.

AFTERWORD

REMEMBER THIS!

Your health isn't determined by luck—it's the result of the choices you make every day. Over time, those choices add up, shaping whether you live with vitality or face illness.

This book has armed you with the knowledge and tools to make healthier decisions, all grounded in the latest scientific research. Change takes time, and there's no quick fix for sustainable health. But every small step you take today leads to big rewards tomorrow—more energy, more milestones to celebrate, and a longer, more fulfilling life.

One of the greatest truths about health is that it often feels invisible. It's the silent foundation that enables you to enjoy life without limits. Only when it's gone do you realize how essential it was. Sadly, the signs of an unhealthy lifestyle often show up too late, in illness or premature loss of life.

Putting off a lifestyle change may feel easier in the moment, but it only makes the journey harder later.

As mentioned at the beginning of this book, every decision has a consequence—even the decision to do nothing.

- Good luck, and may health be with you -

/ Magnus

If you are interested in updates on the book or when there is a new release you can sign-up to get an email on this.

ABOUT THE AUTHOR

My name is Magnus Bengtsson and I am a trained nurse and I'm from Sweden. For many years I worked in the pharmaceutical industry, the Medtech industry and finally in the eHealth industry.

This is my story and background why I wrote 'The Complete Guide to Sustainable Health and Weight'.

Simply put - 2012 could have been my last year. Too early if you ask me. It started with me experiencing strange back pains with physical exertion. I consulted a surgeon who found an issue on xray in my back but which causes absolutely no back pain. 'Have you had your heart checked?' he asked.

I had high cholesterol which my GP somewhat nonchalantly thought I could continue to treat with Omega-3. You want to trust your doctor but unfortunately you can't always do that. You have to be healthy sceptic. If you have no knowledge of medicine, however, it is difficult. With this guide I want to help you to get that.

In the end, I did a health check including an exercise ECG. Thankfully, the doctor who performed the test was a specialist in cardiology. He observed a change on the ECG at maximum load. He therefore referred me to the cardiology department, which, after a number of further tests, referred me for a coronary angiography, i.e. a contrast X-ray of the heart's vessels.

It showed a narrowing that was treated with balloon dilatation and a so-called stent was placed in the vessel. I could have been satisfied with that and continued living as before.

But I wanted the best possible health outcome. It is my life that is at stake. To the medical community, I'm really just a number in the statistics. Dead or alive. If I die, absolutely no one in the healthcare system will find it as sad as I find it myself. For me, it was obvious that I had to take control of my life. And the solution to that is - KNOWLEDGE.

To be clear - in the choice between being healthy, living a long life and being able to do what I want to do when I retire or becoming a young obituary, it was a no brainer for me. It's also a no brainer that I'd have to change my way of life to get that outcome. And if YOUR health is at stake, you need to do exactly that - CHANGE YOUR LIFESTYLE.

I looked at what science had concluded about the effects of diet, exercise, etc. on health risk factors. And the vast majority of studies pointed out that a diet consisting mostly of plant-based foods is best for the heart and also for reducing the risk of other diseases such as cancer. And new evidence on what is good and bad for our health is published every week. The knowledge I learnt initially I have gradually built on over the last 4 years. And I want to share it with you so that you don't end up in the same situation as I did.

In 2020, I started subscribing to newsletters from medical journals to get the latest science on diet, exercise, lifestyle, obesity. As a result, I started the website Forskning | Hälsa where I publish new translated and summarized studies ongoing. In the autumn of 2024 I've published over 300 studies and reports.

In this guide, I have summarized the most important and most recently published studies and added information from various authorities.

You will also find a behavioral science model on how to change your lifestyle in a sustainable way to lose weight.

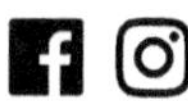